Behind the Pink Ribbon
written by: Melissa Ann Adams

FOREWORD

We had matching pink shirts and tutus and waited nervously at the start line of a half marathon. It was a first for both of us. I couldn't help but tear up as I thought of how much this moment meant to be running in honor of Cancer Fighting Princess. In my mind I was thinking of how wonderful it was to share in such a triumph over cancer by running 13 miles, and also thought of all of the amazing young women that I had met who were too ill to accomplish such a feat or those whose earthly journey was cut short by breast cancer. Melissa is someone who started as a patient but has become a friend as well. I was really honored to share this moment with her.

While breast cancer is the most common cancer in women, affecting one in 8 women in their lifetime, breast cancer in young women is thankfully rare. The risk to develop breast cancer is one in over 19,000 at age 25, one in over 2,500 at age 30, but sharply decreases to one in just over 200 by age 40. Although uncommon, breast cancer in young women is frequently more aggressive and carries a higher mortality. With some types of cancers, reaching the 5-year mark after diagnosis is synonymous with cure. In breast cancer however, particularly breast cancers that express hormone receptors, there can be late recurrences as well as the development of new breast cancers with time. Indeed, recently the medicine tamoxifen has been shown to help prevent some of these late recurrences, when taken for 10 years instead of the traditional 5 years. This benefit is seen particularly in years 10-14 after diagnosis. As such, breast cancer is not just a passing inconvenience to young women who have suffered with it, but it becomes a long and pervasive battle.

The care of young women with breast cancer is a unique situation and in these circumstances a number of additional issues must be considered. Treatment options, side effects and outcomes are discussed with patients of all ages. But to those young women, particularly those in their 20's and 30's, there are a number of challenges that can take on greater significance. The body image issues can be greater. Younger women have concerns about fertility, more long term or late complications of treatment, and the effects of the therapies on their young families and blossoming careers. Many times, in clinical trials, seven year or ten year data is presented. Both my patients and myself, however, hope to think in much longer time frames. Not just what is a chance of a particular side effect developing in the next ten years, but importantly, how likely will that patient live to see their grandchildren 40 years from now?

Being an oncologist that specializes in breast cancer is challenging and rewarding, intellectually stimulating and emotionally intense. The highs, like telling someone they had a complete response to chemotherapy, which is strongly correlated with cure, are awesome, but the lows like having an end of life discussion with a 35 year old with 2 little kids are heartbreaking. I can particularly identify with these young women, as I am a young woman myself. When I have a patient who has children the same age as mine, who is arranging her chemo schedule to see the first day of school send off, as I am arranging my clinic schedule to do the same for my own children, their journey really hits home. When I was pregnant with my now 7-year-old twins and in fellowship training, I had a patient who was pregnant with twins too. She was recently diagnosed with breast cancer and needed to undergo chemotherapy while she was pregnant. I knew as I was going over the side effects of her chemotherapy regimen that she was thinking about her babies. As future moms, we both already knew that we were not just thinking about ourselves anymore. As an oncologist, I can give statistics, and I can share anecdotes of other patients' experiences, but I know that each woman will have their own, unique journey. I am lucky to learn from and share in these journeys, too.

With a new breast cancer diagnosis, many hope that this will be like getting a gallbladder or appendix removed. But soon it becomes evident that the scars, both physically and mentally will linger much longer. As Melissa so eloquently and passionately describes her circumstances, she allows her readers to experience the raw emotion associated with this disease. Not only in the acute phase of treatment, but in the years that follow. How one can move forward while looking over your shoulder? I think this should be required reading for all young women in a similar situation and all those who are part of their lives. This includes their friends and relatives and importantly their medical team, as well. I thank the many women, including Melissa, who have trusted me to be their physician and allowed me to participate in a reciprocal relationship of learning and friendship.

Shannon Puhalla, MD
Director of Breast Cancer Clinical Research at University of Pittsburgh

ACKNOWLEDGEMENTS

First and foremost, thank you to my parents, Kathy and Phil, my grandmother, Anna Mae (may she rest in peace), my great Aunt Aggie, my brothers, Jay and Philip, my sister-in-law, Roxanne, my three amazing nieces, Victoria, Caitlin, and Calie, and my cousins, Dina and Dennis, for being my biggest cheerleaders in all of this. It was your strength, love and support, that got me through the darkest of days.

Thank you to my medical team at UPMC, Pittsburgh - Dr. Gretchen Ahrendt, Dr. Shannon Puhulla, Dr. Michael Gimbel, Dr. Sushil Beriwal, Dr. Kristen Zorn - for your knowledge and skill to treat and heal my body. Thank you for your gentleness and patience when I came unraveled, when I questioned everything, and when I didn't always comply with your recommendations. Thank you to my amazing nurses- Barb, Linda, Judy, and Diane- for wiping away my tears, holding my hand when I needed a gentle touch, all of the hugs, cheering me on, and loving on me like I was your own daughter.

Thank you to all of my friends who were there in many different ways to help me through this journey. Your love and support will always be cherished. I have to give a huge shout out to my friend, Annette, who stepped in and helped in every way possible from taking me to appointments, being at some of my procedures, taking me to get my hair washed, taking out my trash, having her new boyfriend push me in a breast cancer race through the hills of Pittsburgh, and for being my primary caregiver. A million thank you's will never be enough to express the gratitude I have in my heart for you.

Thank you to my husband, Bud, for stepping into the beautiful disaster that I called my life at a time when I needed you the most. Thank you for falling in love with me, as Melissa. You taught me that unconditional love truly exists and despite all of the baggage and the scars that I carry with me, I am still lovable and worthy. You taught me how to love myself again when I never thought I would. And of course, thank you for making it possible for me to meet one of my man crushes- Gavin Rossdale.

Thank you to my dragon boat coach, Lynne, for helping me to find my place in the world again. You never treated me like I had cancer and never allowed me to use that as an excuse for not showing up and doing the work. You pushed me harder than anyone else has ever pushed me before in my life. You made me believe in myself again. You taught me everything that I know about coaching and dragon boating so that I am now able to pay that forward to my own team.

Thank you to Lori and Jeffri-Lynn for taking the time to read my book and offering feedback on edits.

Thank you to my personal coach, Christina, for pushing me to finally get out of my own way and publish this book.

INTRODUCTION

"Give it one year. All of this will be over and behind you. You can go back to normal." I wish I could remember who had said that to me early on in my diagnosis of breast cancer. I held onto those words like it was the gospel. Reality hit me, when a year later, my journey wasn't over, it wasn't behind me, and things sure as hell weren't ever going back to normal. In fact, year after year, for 6 more years, it wasn't over and it wasn't behind me, and I realized that I didn't even know what "normal" was. For 7 years of my life, it seemed as though dealing with cancer-related surgeries, treatment, and issues seemed to be my new normal.

In March 2007, I was diagnosed with genetic invasive ductal carcinoma-breast cancer. I was 31 years old. I did not find my lump through a self-breast exam, a mammogram, or even an exam at my gynecologist's office. In fact, I had just been to the gynecologist about 6 months prior and got a clean report on the breast exam. I just happened to touch my right breast in the exact location where this lump seemed to take up residency but I never thought it was cancer.

I called for an appointment with the gynecologist but was told to wait a week to see if it disappeared. It didn't. When I saw the gynecologist, he told me that it certainly wasn't cancer, that I was too young, and that I need not worry about the family history of cancer on the paternal side of my family. He was wrong.

I never heard the doctor tell me that I had cancer. I only heard her say, "I don't know how to tell you this over the phone". I was devastated. My world came to a screeching halt. It took my breath away. All I could do was tuck my head between my legs for fear of passing out but was also screaming loud enough that my co-workers came rushing into my office.

The days, weeks, and months after my diagnosis were a bit of blur. Navigating the cancer world means appointment after appointment after appointment. It means putting everything else in your life on hold in an attempt to save your life. It means learning about medical terminology. It means trying to understand what you are being told while also trying to process it quickly and make potentially life-saving decisions all at the same time. It means having to rely on family and friends in a way that you never expected, and hoping they show up. It means finding a new normal because the life you had pre-cancer becomes a different life.

I started writing my journal for myself and my closest family and friends. I didn't have the energy to repeat myself over and over to everyone that wanted to know what happened at each appointment. I love that so many people cared so much for me but it was mentally and emotionally exhausting. Journaling became a format for me to express myself when I could not do it verbally. It became an outlet for me to be truthful about my experience and my feelings, rather than trying to hide the reality of it. It was cathartic.

In my journal, I share all the details of my cancer journey from finding my lump, getting the diagnosis, doctor's appointments, surgeries, dealing with my emotions, trying to deal with other people's emotions, becoming a voice for young women with breast cancer, searching for my new normal, dating while dealing with cancer, and even finding love.

In sharing my story, my hope is that anyone touched by breast cancer-survivors, caregivers, supporters, and even doctors, gain a deeper understanding of the reality that sits behind the pink ribbon. Every story of breast cancer is different and not everyone experiences the same course of treatment, the same level of support, the same emotions, or even the same outcome. If my story helps to inspire and give hope to at least one person, it will have been worth all of the hard work of putting this book together.

Much Love!

Tuesday, February 20, 2007
Discovery Day

I just returned from my annual trip to Edinboro for President's Day weekend. As I was putting my makeup on this morning, I couldn't remember if I had brought back the pair of shoes that I needed for today. I got up to look in the bottom of my closet for the shoes and as I was standing back up, I put my left hand on my right breast and felt something unusual - a lump. I stopped dead in my tracks with a million different thoughts rushing through my head but didn't feel a sense of immediate panic. I hurriedly took my hand off it but then, for some reason, touched it again to see if it was still there. Sure enough, it was. I didn't fret over it too much. I continued to get ready, went to work, and started my day, but then thoughts of what it could be started to consume my mind. I mentioned it to a fellow school psychologist in confidence who encouraged me to call my gynecologist. I haven't even told my parents or closest friends yet. Does she think it can possibly be cancer? I don't believe that it could be. Certainly, it can't be! After much hesitation and thinking about it throughout the afternoon, I finally made the phone call, and the nurse asked if I was having my period. As a matter of fact, I am. Good, that explains the lump.... nothing to be concerned about. She told me to wait a week and call back if the lump does not go away when my period ends.

1

Tuesday, February 27, 2007
Gynecologist Appointment

A week later, the lump continues to exist. I swear I have touched it a thousand times over the last week to see if it is still there. It feels like I have a marble in my boob. It is small and hard like a marble and doesn't move very much but doesn't hurt at all. I called my gynecologist's office to let them know that the lump was still there. They asked to see me later today for an exam. I usually am very fussy about seeing male gynecologists, but there wasn't anyone else in today to do the breast exam. When I went in for the exam, the gynecologist, Dr. Robert Thomas, seemed surprised that I am only 31. He asked me several questions about my family history of cancer. I shared with him, as I have with so many others before him, that my paternal grandmother died from ovarian cancer and that my paternal uncle is currently battling prostate cancer. I don't know many details other than that because I don't have any contact with that side of my family. He seemed unconcerned, like the others, that it could be cancer. He told me that my grandmother was too distant from me for me to be concerned. That surprised me. She is my grandmother; she is not too distant! Though Dr. Thomas continued to say that he doubted it was cancer, he recommended I go for a diagnostic mammogram and ultrasound to be on the safe side. I left the office feeling pretty good that this lump is nothing of concern. I mean, after all, he is a doctor and has probably seen this time and time again, and I am sure he knows when something is cancer and when it is not. He said that I can go to St. Margaret Hospital, which is 2 minutes from my apartment, or I can go to Magee Women's Hospital, which is about 30 minutes. Since Dr. Thomas is convinced that there isn't much to be concerned about, I opted for St. Margaret. There is no sense in driving all the way to Oakland when no one seems to be overly worried that it is cancer.

Friday, March 2, 2007
Mammogram/ultrasound

It seems like today took forever to get here. I'm becoming somewhat obsessed with the idea that it could be cancer. I have spent many sleepless nights since I saw my gynecologist searching for information on the Internet. This may not necessarily be the best idea. I showed up for my appointment today only to find out that I was a WEEK early for my appointment! I was so completely distraught and was on the verge of tears. I begged and pleaded with the nurses to find a way to squeeze me in today. It was only 2 pm, and they were booked until 4 but said they would take me if I could wait that long. I agreed and went to my car to get my laptop so that I could at least do some work while I sat there. It was creepy being in that office. I was clearly the youngest person in there by probably 25 to 30 years. I felt like everyone was looking at me saying, "Why is SHE here?" It was very awkward, but I sat and worked until they finally called me back for the mammogram.

I got undressed from the waist up and sat in the hallway while waiting for someone to tell me what to do next. A nurse took me into an exam room where she completed the mammogram. She told me to place my boob on the plate and hold on to the bar. She also told me not to breathe...what? What do you mean I cannot breathe? That is just silly. I continued breathing despite her instructions and endured the pain as she squished my breasts in the machine. She asked me to wait in the hallway while she consulted with the radiologist. I sat there looking around for something to do and found a pamphlet on breast cancer...as if I haven't already read enough on the topic. The nurse returned after a few minutes and said that I need to have another mammogram to get a different perspective, so back in I went to repeat what we had already done. She once again asked me to sit and wait while she spoke with the radiologist. At this point, I was getting utterly bored with this process. But once again, she came back out and told me that I needed to get another one! Come on...surely there is no need for this. We went back into the exam room. As we were ready to start the third mammogram, the radiologist came into the room. The radiologist, Dr. Kanek, said there was no need to do another one and asked that I be escorted over to the waiting area to have the ultrasound.

I grabbed my belongings and walked through the hallway with my hospital gown that could have fit about ten of me and sat in the waiting room for a half-hour before I was called back for the ultrasound. I laid down on the table and let the ultrasound technician view both of my breasts with her little wand. Too bad it wasn't a magic wand and make whatever this lump is disappear. I was able to view the monitor from the table and clearly saw the difference between the right and left breasts. There were a ton of little white specs on the right side, but the left side had none. Well, that can't be good. She saw the concern in my face, and though I knew she couldn't tell me anything, I still asked what she thought it could be. She smiled at me politely and said she wasn't sure. I'm convinced that she knew what it is exactly but was not allowed to tell me. After a few minutes, the radiologist came into the room. This scared me because of all the times I had to go for ultrasound/sonograms (due to ovarian cysts), I have never had a radiologist come into the room during or after the exam. At this point, I feared the worst. Dr. Kanek told me that I have zero fat in my breast area, making it difficult to see, but she thought it imperative that I schedule a biopsy as soon as possible. She said that my gynecologist's office would have the results of the mammogram and ultrasound by Wednesday of next week.

Monday, March 5, 2007
Mammogram/Ultrasound Results

I received a phone call at work from my gynecologist's office that they had the results of the mammogram and the ultrasound. Hmm...that was much faster than what the radiologist told me it would be, but I was feeling relieved that I may have answers soon. Then they said I need to go for an ultrasound-guided fine-needle aspiration of the lump, which they scheduled for the following Monday. Ugh...another week of waiting and wondering! The nurse told me that I would not be permitted to drive myself home from this procedure, so I need to plan to have someone with me. Up to this point, I have not told any of my family or friends that I found a lump and that I had the preliminary tests. My Uncle Tony (my step dad's brother) passed away in August of 2006, and we recently found out that my aunt (my step dad's sister) has cancer too. Now I have to drop this bomb on them! I called them when I got home from work to let them know that I needed to go for a biopsy to exam a lump that I found in my breast. I tried to make it sound as routine as possible in hopes that they wouldn't get upset. I called my Aunt Aggie to tell her as well and ask if she would go with me to the appointment. She, of course, agreed. Another week of waiting, sleepless nights, and searching the Internet...I hope this ends soon!

Monday, March 12, 2007
Biopsy

I went to work for a half-day today because sitting in the apartment all morning was not a good idea, as I know my mind would wander. I finally shared with my other co-workers that I had gone through some preliminary tests and that I would be going for the biopsy. To my surprise and complete dismay, the co-worker I initially told about the lump took it upon herself to tell the entire office about my lump and also made a comment that I was blowing all of this out of proportion! I was outraged, to say the least, but didn't say anything because right now I need to focus on me. I met my Aunt Aggie at my apartment around 11am, and we went to St. Margaret. I decided to go there instead of going to Magee since I don't think it can be cancer. I was fidgeting like a little kid in the waiting room...I didn't know what to do with myself.

They told me that the biopsy would take approximately a half-hour and that I wouldn't feel anything because they would use a local anesthetic. Nothing could have been further from the truth. When I was called back, I asked that my aunt wait in the waiting area and not come with me during the biopsy. They took me into a room that I thought for sure was a closet, but it was actually the exam room. Five medical staff members were around me as I lay on the table during the biopsy. They covered me with a warm blanket because I was shivering. When Dr. Kanek entered the room, she stood above my head and repeatedly told me what a beautiful, young woman I am and how everything will be fine. By the way that they were treating me, I started to become convinced that they thought for sure it was cancer. Dr. Kanek then explained that she would numb the breast area to make a small incision to extract tissue from the tumor. I have never had a local anesthetic before, but I know from my experience today, it did not work.

I felt everything she did- all 7 times that she went in to extract tissue, when the anesthesia was administered and re-administered, and when a small metallic chip was inserted to identify the site of the tumor. The biopsy took almost 2 hours, and I almost passed out twice. When she extracted tissue, it took everything in me not to jump off the table. I would imagine the only thing that might feel the same would be getting shot at point-blank range. I sobbed throughout the entire procedure. They had to stop several times because I was crying so hard. I became very nauseous and almost passed out about the 4th or 5th time she inserted the needle. They had to stop and put a cold compress on my head for a few minutes. Dr. Kanek stroked my hair and told me how sorry she is that I had to be doing this and that it broke her heart because I looked like a baby doll lying there on the table. She asked me if I was okay to continue, and when I was ready, she proceeded with the extraction. Once finished, a nurse stood over me for about fifteen minutes putting heavy, constant pressure on the incision. Dr. Kanek was concerned because I had zero fat tissue, so she suspected it would be harder for the bleeding to stop. She was right. I was sobbing and wanted it to end. Dr. Kanek tried to soothe me by stroking my hair and telling me it was going to be okay. "We are going to fight this," she said. I regained my composure and started to get dressed. As I did, they brought my Aunt Aggie back. She could tell that I was totally exhausted from the procedure. Dr. Kanek said my gynecologist would have the results of the biopsy soon, but I might want to call on Wednesday to schedule an appointment. As my aunt and I were leaving, Dr. Kanek pulled us into her office and continued to assure me that things would be fine. She told me once again how young and beautiful I am, and that they will do everything they can to get me through this. I was taken aback by her words and wasn't sure what to make of it. Was she trying to tell me that I have breast cancer without really telling me? Or could it be something else? I don't know, but I was also in so much pain that I couldn't even begin to think about the possibilities. My aunt took me home and stayed with me for about 5 hours. I fell in and out of sleep several times. I had to put pressure on the incision site to stop the bleeding, but 6 hours later, I was still bleeding. I called Dr. Kanek at home (she gave me her number just in case), and she told me I could go to the emergency room where they would only have me sit with someone standing over me applying pressure. I wasn't feeling well and didn't want to go to the emergency room to have someone do what I could do myself. My aunt left, and I laid on the chaise for a long time in quite a daze. I cuddled with my cat, Princess Bailey Head, for most of the evening. I can't believe this is happening to me. I don't want to get up tomorrow and go to work!

Wednesday, March 14, 2007
Scheduling

I called my gynecologist's office today to schedule an appointment to get the results of the biopsy. I was told that Dr. Thomas was not in and would not be in until the end of the week. I explained that I needed to come into the office as soon as possible to get the results. I was simply told that someone would be in touch with me to schedule an appointment once Dr. Thomas returned.

Thursday, March 15, 2007
Diagnosis Day

I was in my office for about a half-hour when my phone rang. The lady on the other end of the line identified herself. I didn't know who she was but assumed she was the parent of a student I am evaluating or was calling to request a special education evaluation for her child. We have many doctors that reside within the school district where I work. Once she realized that I thought this was a work-related phone call rather than a personal phone call, she identified herself as one of the doctors from my gynecologist's office. I thought she was going to ask me to come in to review the results of my biopsy since I had called yesterday asking for an appointment. Instead, all I heard her say was, "I don't know how to tell you this over the phone"...I never heard anything more than that. I started screaming for one of the secretaries in my office. I don't know how loud I was because everything was so hazy. Someone came running into my office and saw that I was sitting there with my head tucked between my legs screaming and crying with the phone in my hand but not to my ear. She took the phone from me and talked to the doctor. I don't know how long I sat there with my head between my legs...it seemed like forever. I know that eventually, three of my coworkers, Naomi, Cindy, and Cathy, were all kneeling on the floor in front of me, and I was crying and shaking uncontrollably.

I wanted to call my dad but couldn't recall his phone number. Go figure that I forgot my cell phone at home. I tried calling my aunt, but she wasn't at home. Cindy drove me to my apartment to get my cell phone, so I could call my dad. I think he was as shocked as I was because he only said, "That sucks." I said, "Yeah, I know. It's like a kick in the balls." After talking to him, I called my friend Kathy in Erie and told her. She was trying so hard not to cry, but I knew that she was. I went back to work but didn't do very much. I had meetings scheduled but wasn't in the right frame of mind to go.

I emailed some of my friends at work and asked them to call me so I could share the news. When my best friend came to my office, it took everything in me to hold it together when I told him. The look of devastation on his face will forever be etched in my mind. I honestly have no idea what I did for the rest of the day. It was so surreal. I was so angry at that doctor because I had called for an appointment. I knew it was cancer and didn't want to be at work when I got the news. I was so pissed for never having that option. I came home tonight and took out the pink ribbon pin that the pharmacist at the Edinboro Giant Eagle grocery store gave me about 3 years ago and made the promise to myself to wear a pink ribbon every day.

Wednesday, March 21, 2007
Surgical Oncologist / Geneticist / MRI

My mom, Aunt Aggie, and I went to my first doctor's appointment since being diagnosed. Dr. Gretchen Ahrendt, my surgical oncologist, entered the exam room and had tears in her eyes before she even saw me. She examined me, explained the mammogram to me, and answered some of the questions that I had about what I had read about breast cancer. Dr. Ahrendt requested that my mom and Aunt Aggie come into the room. She explained to them that I have Invasive Ductal Carcinoma and Ductal Carcinoma In-Situ (DCIS). I have a large cluster of DCIS around the tumor and some in outlying areas. Dr. Ahrendt is recommending that I undergo a mastectomy.

Dr. Ahrendt inquired about my family history, which my mom shared with her. I had no idea that there was such a strong paternal history of cancer. She recommended that I have genetic testing and an MRI done, which she was able to schedule for today. I left her office feeling kind of numb knowing that I will be losing a part of me. I didn't say much during the remaining 4-5 hours that we were there. What was there to say? I completed part of the genetic testing process, which consisted of developing a family tree on both sides of my family. The geneticist shared with me the implications of having a gene mutation. I then went for the MRI, which was a unique experience. They put an IV in me and then injected something that made my mouth taste like saltwater. I had to lie down in the machine face down. It was uncomfortable, and I had to stay completely still for a half-hour. They also injected something that made me feel like I peed my pants. When I was done, they took the IV out of my arm, and I bled horribly; the blood was running down my arm. That was really freaky! After the MRI, I returned to the genetics department to have my blood drawn. I despise needles, so being stabbed twice in one day was not fun for me.

Friday, March 23, 2007
MRI Results

Dr. Ahrendt called me to let me know that the MRI confirmed the need for a mastectomy. The tumor is small and low-grade, but the DCIS is larger, scattered, and a higher-grade (faster growing). She scheduled an appointment for me to meet with a plastic surgeon.

I came home that evening, snuggled up on the couch with Princess Bailey Head, and watched Why I Wore Red Lipstick to my Mastectomy. I don't know why I watched it; I was sobbing through the entire movie. I thought it might be helpful since I will be having a mastectomy soon.

Wednesday, April 4, 2007
Plastic Surgeon Consultation

My friend, Jill, and I met with the plastic surgeon, Dr. Michael Gimbel, to talk about my reconstruction options following the mastectomy. Dr. Gimbel examined me and took some photos. He indicated that I have two possible options: the free-tram flap, which would involve using my abdominal fat to reconstruct my breast or implants- either silicone or saline. It was a lot of information to take in and very surreal at times. He said that I'm only a marginal candidate for the free-tram flap procedure, but it seems like the better option in my opinion. With the implants, I would have to undergo several surgeries. I will have to have surgery again down the line because I'm so young and the implants only have a "shelf life" of ten years. There are positives and negatives to each of these options, but I'm not under any significant pressure to make a decision right now, though I'm pretty sure I want the free-tram flap procedure. Dr. Gimbel suggested that I look at some of the pictures of other women that have undergone reconstructive surgery. I tried but couldn't; I broke down into tears as soon as I opened the book.

My surgical oncologist, Dr. Ahrendt, called to schedule several appointments. On Monday, April 9th, I will be having a biopsy of my sentinel lymph node to determine if cancer has spread from the tumor into the lymphatic system. This will help determine the need for radiation before my surgery or after my surgery or at all. It will also determine when the reconstruction can be done, which I'm hoping it can all be done at the same time.

My tentative surgery date is May 3rd (my step dad's birthday! UGH!). Dr. Ahrendt said I will be in the hospital for at least 4 days. Depending on which type of reconstruction I have, I will be laid up for at least a month. This means that I will not be participating in the Race for the Cure on May 13th, but I will be there in spirit.

Thursday, April 5, 2007
I'm a Teenage Mutant Ninja Turtle

I received a phone call from Darcy Thull, a geneticist at the Cancer Genetics Department, today. Results of the testing reveal that I do have a genetic mutation– BRCA2, meaning that I do have an increased chance of developing cancer again in my left breast, as well as in my ovaries. Wow...this week keeps getting better. There are several decisions that I will have to make based on this information, such as opting for a preventive bilateral mastectomy and removal of my ovaries. UGH! Not only does this mutation have implications for me, but also for my family members on the paternal side. My family history is significant for ovarian cancer, breast cancer, colon cancer, and prostate cancer, which are all linked to this genetic mutation. I joked with the geneticist and said that it confirms that I am a Teenage Mutant Ninja Turtle, but deep down, it cut straight through me like a knife. I hung up the phone and cried.

Shortly after talking with the geneticist, Dr. Ahrendt called me to talk about the implications of the BRCA2 mutation. She offered her apologies, which makes it seem so much worse. It feels completely unreal.

Tuesday, April 9, 2007
Sentinel Lymph Node Biopsy

Yesterday I had surgery to remove some of my lymph nodes. I was at Magee from 10 am until 7 pm. My Aunt Aggie took me in, and then my friend Jill came later to be with me and take me home. I got into pre-op at approximately 10:45 am. It was nice because I got to take a nap for a bit. They took me to the breast center to get a dye injection to help my surgeon determine which lymph nodes would most likely be affected by cancer first. I went back to my pre-op room and had to have an IV put in my hand. I hate needles, but the nurse was gentle and numbed my hand before inserting the IV. I got to take another nap before I went into surgery around 1:30 pm.

I had never been into an operating room before - it was an experience. It was all stainless steel, and huge lights were placed over the surgical table– not what I remember seeing in the TV show ER. Anyway, they gave me a gas mask, and within three deep breaths, I was out. The surgery took approximately 45 minutes, but I was sedated for a very long time. I didn't "come to" until about 5 pm. The nurse was making me mad because she was trying to wake me up and took my water away from me. She even put my bed all the way up so that I was pretty much sitting, but that didn't stop me from falling back to sleep. I went to a step-down recovery room at approximately 5:30 or 6 (but my recollection of time is probably a bit off because I was so out of it). My Aunt Aggie and Jill were able to be with me again while I was there. I was still fatigued and wanted to go back to sleep. Finally, I was released at approximately 7 pm. Jill brought me home and put me to bed. She got my prescription for the painkillers filled for me. I stayed in bed all night for the most part, but I got sick at about 10pm. The most important thing is that the preliminary results indicate that cancer has not spread to my lymph nodes. That is some good news... considering.

My arm is still sore today. The incision is relatively large, and I guess it represents my first battle wound. I haven't needed the pain medication...Tylenol has been working just fine. I have to call Dr. Ahrendt, surgical oncologist, in a bit to schedule my follow up appointment with her.

The biggest struggle for me right now is not having control over this and having to lean on everyone else to take care of me. I've always been freakishly independent, and now I can't even shower myself or do my own hair. It is incredibly frustrating, but I'm so thankful to have all of my friends and family to see me through this most trying time.

Tuesday, April 10, 2007
The Best Day of My Life

This poem is from the book Nordie's at Noon that I recently read about four young women (ages 24, 27, 27, and 30) who also battled breast cancer. I enjoyed this poem and wanted to share it. Though each day is a struggle for me, I try to remember this poem:

Today, when I awoke, I suddenly realized that this is the best day of my life, ever! There were times when I wondered if I would make it to today, but I did! And because I did, I'm going to celebrate.

Today, I'm going to celebrate what an unbelievable life I have had so far; the accomplishments, the many blessings, and yes, even the hardships because they have served to make me stronger.

I will go through this day with my head held high, and a happy heart.

I will marvel at God's seemingly simple gifts: the morning dew, the sun, the clouds, the trees, the flowers, the birds. Today, none of these miraculous creations will escape my notice.

Today, I will share my excitement for life with other people. I'll make someone smile. I'll go out of my way to perform an unexpected act of kindness for someone I don't even know.

Today, I'll give a sincere compliment to someone who seems down. I'll tell a child how special he is, and I'll tell someone I love just how deeply I care for them and how much they mean to me.

Today is the day I quit worrying about what I don't have and start being grateful for all the wonderful things God has already given me.

I'll remember that to worry is just a waste of time because my faith in God and his Divine Plan ensures everything will be just fine.

Tonight, before I go to bed, I'll go outside and raise my eyes to the heavens. I will stand in awe at the beauty of the stars and the moon, and I will praise God for these magnificent treasures.

As the day ends and I lay my head down on my pillow, I will thank the Almighty for the best day of my life. And I will sleep the sleep of a contented child, excited with expectation because I know tomorrow is going to be...

THE BEST DAY OF MY LIFE!
~ Gregory M. Lousignont, Ph.D.

Thursday, April 12, 2007
Biopsy Results

Dr. Ahrendt, my surgical oncologist, called me a few minutes ago to let me know that the pathology report indicates that my lymph nodes are clear of cancer, which means that I can undergo reconstruction immediately following surgery and will not have to undergo radiation therapy. I meet with her on April 20th to discuss the implications of the BRCA2 and my options for surgery/reconstruction (i.e., doing the mastectomy on only the right side and monitoring the left side, doing a bilateral mastectomy, and the pros and cons of the reconstruction options, etc.). So at least there was some good news in all of this.

Sunday, April 15, 2007
Facing the Days

Well, this is my first entry to not report on anything from the doctors but an expression of how I feel. The past 2 days have been horrible, and it has taken everything in me to get out of bed. I lay there for hours hoping that if I put my head under the blankets and ignore the fact that my world has been completely shattered, it will all just go away. But it doesn't go away- it is still there. Every second of every minute of every hour of every day, it is there. Because of that, I hate what my life has become. I want to go back to my simple pre-cancer life! I would give anything to have back what was normal for me. But I can't go back, and I hate facing every new day and every new piece of information and every decision that I have to make.

When I found out the cancer is genetic, it was like being handed my death sentence. It is bad enough that I have it already, but to know that I will more than likely get it again on the left side and/or in my ovaries is too much to take. I'm faced with decisions that I'm not ready to make, but I know I can't delay the process. I know that I'm going to be okay because I am determined to be, but that doesn't mean that I'm okay with any of this. I'm not okay with the fact that I have any type of cancer at this age. I'm not okay with the fact that I have to give up a part of who I am as a woman in an attempt to save my life. I'm not okay with having to decide on doing a bilateral mastectomy to try to prevent cancer on the other side. I'm not okay with the fact that there is no suitable method to screen for ovarian cancer. I'm not okay with not knowing that any of this is for sure or that cancer won't come back. I'm not okay with how all of this will impact me in the future with relationships and children. I'm not okay with any of this at all. I am angry, hurt, scared, and I want to scream, cry, and stay in bed. I feel so violated, cheated, and robbed. I feel so broken and damaged in all the ways that define me as a woman.

Thursday, April 19, 2007
Change a life, make a difference, and touch a heart!

On April 8th and April 18th, I presented my story along with some statistics and risk factors of breast cancer to the elementary and high schools that I am assigned to in my district. (Note: I would never in a MILLION years do something like this, but it was an opportunity that I couldn't let slip away.) This is what I shared:

"My name is Melissa Ward. I'm the school psychologist for your school. From a very young age, my goals in life have been to change a life, make a difference, and touch a heart. Well, the opportunity to do just that has presented itself to me in a way that I can't even begin to grasp. But it is real, and I am going to take advantage of that opportunity. On March 15, 2007, I was diagnosed with breast cancer at the age of 31. I was ignorant to the fact that I could have breast cancer at such a young age. It was important for me to come here today to speak to all of you to increase your awareness of breast cancer in young women. As the incidence of young women with breast cancer is much lower than in older women, young women are an underrepresented population in many research studies.

However, statistics* indicate that 1 in 229 women between the ages of 30 and 39 will be diagnosed with breast cancer within the next 10 years. The youngest girl diagnosed with breast cancer in the Pittsburgh area was 13 years old. Breast cancer is the leading cause of cancer death in young women ages 15 to 54. More than 11,000 women under the age of 40 will be diagnosed with breast cancer this year, and more than 1100 will die. Cancer in young women is generally more aggressive and results in lower survival rates. The 5-year survival rate for young women with breast cancer is 82%.

Some of the risk factors* for breast cancer are:

1. Gender- women are 100 times more likely to have breast cancer, but it is also possible for men to have the disease.

2. Genetics- about 5-10% of breast cancers are linked to a genetic mutation. This genetic mutation significantly increases the chance of breast cancer by about 87%, as well as ovarian cancer by approximately 45%.

3. Family history- having a mother or sister with the disease increases the likelihood of breast cancer. There is also a link between breast cancer and a family history of ovarian cancer, prostate cancer, and breast cancer diagnosed under the age of 40. This is typically associated with the genetic mutation.

18

4. Being Caucasian.

5. Having a menstrual period before the age of 12.

6. Not having children or having children after the age of 30.

7. Taking birth control pills.

8. Having 2 to 5 alcoholic drinks daily.

9. Being overweight.

10. Lack of exercise.

11. There may also be a link between smoking and breast cancer.

I encourage all of you to become more aware of your possible risk factors for breast cancer, perform self-examinations, learn your family's medical history, and follow up with your doctor if you find something of concern. Early detection can be a lifesaver."

Information obtained from the American Cancer Society in April 2007.

Friday, April 20, 2007
Sentinel Lymph Node Check Up

I met with Dr. Ahrendt, my surgical oncologist, today for her to check my incision from the sentinel lymph node biopsy, to talk about my treatment options, and to discuss the implications of the BRCA2. I'm not sure what to say because I'm still trying to make sense of all of this. In a few weeks, my body as I know it will change forever. Sometimes I sit there talking to her feeling like I'm having an out of body experience or a nightmare that I wish would end now. I have not yet made a decision on the type of reconstruction or the preventative surgery, but I am still leaning toward the free-tram flap procedure. It is a difficult decision for so many reasons that many will never understand. There is no easy answer. As much as I wish it were as easy as going in and get bigger boobs, that is not what it is about at all. I have come to accept my body the way that God gave it to me. I would give anything in this world to keep my body as it is now, despite the size of my boobs. Now I am being forced to re-live my life as an adolescent and learn to accept a whole new image of myself. I have a hard time thinking about and imagining what that is going to be like...to wake up every day and have a constant reminder of what used to be. I'm not prepared for the trauma that I am about to endure.

I was somewhat taken aback today and, of course, the reality of this disease hit me in the face again when I told Dr. Ahrendt that I'm not okay with any of this but that I know I have to do this to save my life. Her response was, "I can't promise you that this will save your life." Ugh! There it is again...my own mortality staring me straight in the face. My own body is its own worst enemy. I feel like there is a ticking time bomb waiting to go off at any minute. Dr. Ahrendt thinks we still have some time with the ovaries, but I will have to start the screening for that now. She shared the same concerns regarding ovarian cancer. That truly gives me no level of comfort at all, but I most certainly want honesty over anything else.

The implications of BRCA2 go well beyond the here and now. A lot of people have viewed this as something that I need to take care of and be done with. The reality of it is that I will have to worry about cancer for the rest of my life! Everything has changed in the blink of an eye; nothing will ever be the same. I have changed, I will never be the same– both inside and out.

Thursday, April 26, 2007
Decision Day

Yesterday, I met with my plastic surgeon, Dr. Gimbel, to discuss my reconstruction options now that we know I am a BRCA2 carrier and to sign the consent forms for the type of surgery I am electing to have done. All things considered, I think I made the "best" choice, though in my opinion not having cancer would be the BEST! I'm still trying to come to terms with the decision that I have made, so I'm not ready to put it out there yet. We confirmed my surgery date for May 3rd~vomit! (Happy Birthday Dad). I had two pre-surgery appointments today- one for a physical and the other to have lab work done. This makes it all too real for me, and I realize that this is coming much sooner than I want.

I tried putting my head under the blankets thing again today, but it still didn't go away. I would give anything in this world to make it all go away. I hate the way I feel; I hate the way this has completely turned my life upside down; I HATE IT ALL! I'm angry at the world, I'm mad at God, and I'm furious at the biological father that passed on his mutated gene to me. He has had nothing to do with me my entire life, and now my life has been upended because of him. That hardly seems fair to me at all. I'm not looking forward to the days before my surgery, and I'm becoming more anxious about it. For me, that means eating less, sleeping less, and crying more. I'm not ready for this at all. I'm not prepared for the emotional and psychological trauma, and I'm most certainly not ready for the physical trauma that my body is about to endure.

Wednesday, May 2, 2007
I'm Not Ready for This

Here it is...the day before my surgery. It seems so long ago that this journey began on February 20th, but tomorrow has come so much faster than I had anticipated. I have to be at the hospital at 5:45 am, and my surgery is at 7:30 am. I have opted to have a bilateral mastectomy to treat cancer on the right side and to try to prevent it on the left side. Since this is the decision I have made, I have no option for reconstruction other than breast implants, which I have been so opposed to from the beginning. My surgical oncologist will conduct a skin-preserving mastectomy, and then the plastic surgeon will insert the tissue expanders and donated skin. The procedure will take approximately 6-8 hours, and I will be spending at least 2 nights in the hospital.

I'm utterly terrified of what I'm going to look like and feel on the other side of this. I have never been so afraid in my life. I just sit in front of the mirror and stare at myself with nothing on to etch that image into my mind so that it is not lost forever. I want to remember me as me, the way that God had made me. Though I know that my breasts do not define me as who I am, they most certainly do define me as a woman. Losing a part of what defines me as a woman is nothing to be minimized. It is something that unless you have been through it, you will never understand it.

I had to take my sweet kitty, Princess Bailey Head, to my Aunt Aggie's house while I am recovering from my surgery. It breaks my heart that she cannot be here with me as she has been a significant source of comfort. She is so intuitive and knows when I need her to snuggle with me. She is in good hands and will be loved and cared for while she is there.

Friday, May 4, 2007
(Written by my BFF, Ken)

The day for Melissa's surgery has now come and gone. The operation lasted until early afternoon and Melissa was in recovery for only a short time. The doctors report that they are very satisfied with how the surgery went. They were not entirely certain of her release date but felt she may be able to come home earlier than expected.

Melissa was obviously quite groggy and "out of sorts" on the phone ... many of us who know her well would be able to tell little difference. LOL. She still had that ability to let out a little laugh that is so adorable, and she still has that great sense of humor.

Later in the evening on Thursday, it was apparent that the medications were wearing off and the surgery was taking its toll. She was very tired, and she was starting to feel the pain a bit more. Her optimism faced the harsh reality that she should not push herself to get out of the hospital early. She recognizes that the hospital is the best place for her to be comfortable. She was not able to speak long, so the conversation was short.

She sends her best to everyone and has been incredibly touched by the amount of support everyone has shown her. We will continue to pray for her and think about her.

Monday, May 7, 2007
Close the Door When You Leave

I'm doing as well as can be expected. I'm resting comfortably at home with the help of all of my family and friends. Typing isn't that easy, so this will be short because I have another poem I want to share. I do want to say thanks for all the unconditional love and support, as well as the prayers and positive thoughts. It is appreciated more than I can ever verbalize. Thank you!! I will check in as often as I can and as I feel up to it! Much Love!

CLOSE THE DOOR WHEN YOU LEAVE

I never asked you to visit...at least I don't believe I did
Maybe...I don't know
It's so confusing

At any rate, you're a rude guest
You take my energy, rob my sleep, and with a stick
You swirl and distort my dreams

All right; You are here- for now
But understand
There are two places that are forever off limits

You may not tread on my spirit
You may not occupy my soul

I have heard of your visits to others
I know the damage you leave in your path
The wanton disregard for innocence, value, and what some would call fairness

Also, I hear that laughter confuses you; that good food makes you feel bad, and
That nothing causes you more distress than an autumn sunset, the forever blue of a summer sky,
Or the unconditional radiance of a child's smile

Listen and understand
You might pilfer my closets, empty all the drawers, and trash my house
But there are two places forever off limits

You may not tread on my spirit
You may not occupy my soul

24

Do not mistake my nausea, weakness, and pain as signs of your victory
They are simply small dents in the armor I wear to fight you
Instead, look deeply into my eyes

They will once again remind you that there are two places forever off limits

You must not...
May not...
Will not tread on my spirit

You must not...
May not...
Will not occupy my soul

~ Michael Hayes Samuelson
(male breast cancer survivor)

Copyright © 2000 by Michael Hayes Samuelson
Author of "Voices from the Edge: Life Lessons from the Cancer Community"
Longstreet Press

Saturday, May 12, 2007
Surgery Day from My Perspective

This is my first update on anything of real importance regarding cancer. I thought about this for some time and decided that I would include my own perspective of the surgery.

May 3, 2007- Surgery Day. I arrived at the hospital promptly at 5:45 am and beat the rest of my family there. I was taken into pre-op rather quickly without my family. The nurse at the front desk said my family would be brought back to me as soon as they arrived. I waited for what seemed like forever and finally called my dad to see where they were. He said they were in the waiting room and were told that they could not come back to me yet. I told the nurse to please go get my family. Before they arrived, the anesthesia student came to insert my IV. She first tried on the top of my left hand, no luck. Then tried a vein in my left forearm, but still no luck. My family arrived, and I was already in tears from having been stabbed one too many times. She then went to get someone with more experience. They tried at the crook of my left elbow, but again, no luck.

Dr. Ahrendt, my surgical oncologist, arrived. I was crying and asked her to make them stop poking me. The anesthesiologist moved over to the right side. They tried the right hand, but again, no luck. At this point, I was tempted to say, "Okay, we are done. I'm not doing this." Finally, they got an IV in the crook of my right elbow. My parents and aunt were by my side, reassuring me that it was going to be okay and giving me lots of love and kisses. Just before I was getting ready to go, I looked at my mom and saw tears falling down her face. Dr. Ahrendt quickly took her out of the room so that I wouldn't see her crying. The look on her face was of pure terror and heartache that her 31year old daughter has cancer and is undergoing major surgery. I wanted to hug her and tell her that it would be okay; that's me being strong for everyone else in my time of need. The last thing I remember was being given something through my IV– something special just for me. I only remember that within a split second, I was in "la-la land." My family told me I had the biggest smile on my face as they wheeled me to surgery. Obviously, I don't recall much after that. The whole process took several hours, from 7:30 am to sometime in the afternoon. I remember waking up in the recovery room and seeing the nurse that had worked with me during my sentinel lymph node biopsy. I said, "And, where were you this morning when they kept stabbing me?" She laughed. Several times in the recovery room, I heard them saying that I have a history of depression. Finally, after about the 4th time, I yelled, "I do not have a history of depression. Get that off my chart."

After a while, two men came to take me to my room. When we got there, I had to move myself from one bed to the next. I hurt like hell, and you want me to move by myself? But I did, and then they helped to straighten me up on the bed. Shortly after, my family was permitted to join me, or maybe they were already there. I don't remember. I had 2 IVs in me now...one for fluids and one for the morphine and anti-nausea meds.

I can't recall much of the evening, but apparently, I was a barrel of laughs for my family, which is what I would have preferred. I do remember asking if I could say something at one point, and they all agreed that I could. They thought it was going to be something profound, I think. I loudly blurted out, "FUCK!!!!" They all looked at me with surprise and laughed. I got sick very little, but dry heaved quite a bit. What did come up was black and freaked me out. I started crying and telling everyone how much I hated this. Then when I was done, I wanted my mouthwash to rinse it out. Can you believe that they didn't give it to me? How rude. After I got sick, the nurse gave me some more anti-nausea medication that knocked me completely out. I remember coming to again and seeing my cousin who had been there for some time and saying, "Hi Dina!" like she just got there. I talked to my friend on the phone for a bit and apparently told him, "If I'm a good little girl, they are going to parole me tomorrow." After visiting hours were over, they kicked everyone out, but let my mom spend the night with me. I was very itchy and asked my dad to get a mechanical pencil from my overnight bag to scratch my stomach and face. Then I saw my sister-in-law had nails like cat claws and made her scratch my stomach and face.

In the morning, I was told that I might be discharged that day or the next, depending on how I felt. Shortly after, the nurse told me I was discharged. Hmm, wasn't all too sure about that. I ordered breakfast, had the catheter and IVs removed, and got washed up. I sat in the chair for several hours and then ordered lunch, including my favorite dessert, carrot cake. At about 2 pm, I decided I was ready to be discharged. I got home at approximately 3 pm. It felt so good to be home!

My dad stayed the night with me. When we woke in the morning, he left to get coffee, and I tried to give myself a sponge bath. When I undressed, I noticed blood on my surgical bra at my incision site for the drain. I immediately called Dr. Ahrendt. She suggested that we go to the emergency room. I called my dad, and he returned to my apartment in a panic. I swear he drove like he was in the Indy 500. Thankfully, I was taken back immediately to be seen. They discovered that my drain was loose. They readjusted it and sent me on my way.

Saturday, May 9, 2007
Post-Op Appointments

I went to see both my plastic surgeon, Dr. Gimbel, and my surgical oncologist, Dr. Ahrendt, yesterday. My first appointment was with Dr. Gimbel to find out if I was ready to have the drains taken out and for him to check the incisions. My sister-in-law took me to my appointment. I didn't even get through the waiting room or the visit without crying this time. I sat there with tears falling down my face and don't even know why. During the appointment, Dr. Gimbel told me that my drains were not ready to come out yet but should be okay by Friday. In his opinion, the incisions looked good, and he pulled off the transparent, sticky dressing. Dr. Gimbel asked if I had looked yet, and I told him that I had not. He said that most people look by now, but I am not ready to look. Dr. Gimbel indicated that we would begin filling the tissue expanders in about two weeks. Within about two and a half months from that time, he would complete another surgery to remove the tissue expanders and replace them with the implants.

I went immediately to meet with Dr. Ahrendt. She, too, looked at my incisions and was pleased with them. She was surprised to see the amount of volume that Dr. Gimbel had put in the tissue expander considering that I have no body fat. She talked to me again about the pathology report. During the surgery, she had the pathologist test the tissue around the tumor, and the margins were not clear. Dr. Ahrendt had to go back in and take out more tissue down toward my upper abs to get a clean margin, which apparently is rather unusual. She had indicated that she would be presenting my case to the breast cancer conference the following evening to determine if the team felt that radiation would be needed since the DCIS (ductal carcinoma in situ- cancer that is still in the milk ducts and non-invasive) was so close to the margins. She talked to me about the possibility of chemotherapy and the factors that help the medical oncologist make that determination. Dr. Ahrendt felt that doing an Oncotype DX test would be beneficial in my case to help make the decision regarding the need for chemotherapy. Despite my not wanting to talk about the removal of my ovaries, she indicated that I would need to do some serious thinking about preserving my eggs if I have to have chemo since my ovaries may not function the same afterward.

Ugh...more decisions that I'm not ready to make. Dr. Ahrendt is also recommending that I begin physical therapy in three weeks to increase my range of motion, especially since I have a vein in my armpit that got caught up in the scar tissue when the sentinel lymph node biopsy was completed and now that vein is very tight, decreasing my range of motion.

I meet with the medical oncologist on June 4th to discuss chemotherapy.

Saturday, May 12, 2007
Drains Removed

I went back to see Dr. Gimbel yesterday. As I got ready in the morning, I decided that it would be the day I finally looked at the reconstruction. I undid the Velcro on my bra and looked in complete shock of what was before me. I will spare you the details of what I saw, but I stood there in complete awe, looking at what used to be my breasts. What I now have are these ugly foreign objects that have indentations. I could only stand there and cry at what I saw before me, knowing that I can't go and undo what has been done.

I actually made it through my first appointment with Dr. Gimbel without crying. WOO HOO! He thought that was great too. I told him that I finally looked at my reconstruction and he asked me what I thought. I told him, "they are ugly," and that was the end of that conversation. He took out the drains...finally, some relief. It didn't hurt when he removed the drains, but it felt weird. He told me that I'm still not permitted to sleep on my side, but I can start exercising the lower half of my body. I brought up the possibility that I might need radiation because I knew that would have implications for his part in all of this. Typically, they try to avoid doing the reconstruction until after someone has had radiation, and that is why the sentinel lymph node biopsy was completed. Dr. Gimbel said that sometimes it does happen that someone may need radiation after they have already begun the reconstruction process. It might be possible that I would have to have another surgery to move healthy muscle tissue to the area where they do the radiation since it will be concentrated in the area close to my upper abs. Ugh...not what I was looking forward to hearing, but I smiled and said, "Okay."

My surgical oncologist, Dr. Ahrendt, called me about an hour after my appointment and told me that after discussing my case last evening, the radiation oncologist feels that it would be necessary for me to have radiation. She also explained in more detail that after radiation, I may need to have muscle tissue moved from my back to the area where the radiation is completed. She indicated that it is not anything that can be determined until after I go through the radiation. Dr. Ahrendt also stated that the medical oncologist suggested that I have the Oncotype DX testing to help make appropriate and informed decisions regarding my need for chemotherapy.

I'm not too sure what I think about all of this. I'm still taking it all in...I feel like my body keeps betraying me and that I'm taking steps backward instead of forward. It feels like this will never be over, and in some way, it never will. No matter how strong and healthy I come out on the other side of this, it will always be there. I have two constant reminders that will always be there.

Monday, May 14, 2007
Cancer Teaches Life Lessons

I can't sleep, the tears keep falling, I'm mourning my loss(es), and I'm feeling rejected. Life is funny...so unpredictable. I have been involved with the breast cancer walks for some time, and the ovarian cancer walk since I found out that my grandmother died from it. Isn't it ironic how the two causes so close to my heart have now become the harsh reality of my own life? Today was the Race for the Cure, and I can't even begin to explain how it felt to be on the other side, sporting my Pink Survivor shirt. It was uplifting and heartbreaking all at the same time. It gave me hope to see all of those women who have battled this same disease, but it broke my heart seeing all of the walkers with "In Memory Of" tags on the back of their shirts. I couldn't help but think that one day someone may be walking with a tag "In Memory Of" me. I know that it won't be anytime soon because I will fight like hell until that day, but the unknown is terrifying and facing your own mortality every day at the age of 31 is something that I can't even begin to explain.

I have learned so many valuable lessons in the short time since my diagnosis. I have learned that every breast cancer patient is different, that no two share the same story. Even with all of the support in the world, there are still days that I feel so alone (listen to Dierks Bentley's Long Trip Alone, that's how I am feeling).

People find strength in different ways. I find mine through my sense of humor and sharing my story in hopes that I can make a difference or change a life.

Not everyone is sincere when they say that they will see me through this to the end; some will drift away and disappear altogether.

 I'm entitled to feel the way I do and don't have to explain why I feel a certain way. It is okay to cry and put my head under the blankets for a while, but then I have to get up and face the day.

People may be insensitive due to ignorance or a lack of understanding, but that doesn't mean it is okay. I love and appreciate those people in my life that will walk side by side with me the whole way so much more.

Saying fuck is a method of therapy. I don't have to like/love my "new" body, but I have to accept it for what it is because I have life. I will come out on the other side of this and turn it into something positive!

They say that when life hands you lemons, make lemonade...my question is, "what if I don't like or want lemonade?" I shouldn't have ever been forced into having to make lemonade instead of a margarita!

30

Tuesday, May 22, 2007
After the rain...the rainbow

I was inspired by someone this evening after having a discussion about rainbows. It made me realize that to see the rainbow, the rain must come first. I guess that my journey through the cancer world is my rain and I will be looking for that rainbow when the rain has stopped...or maybe just slows down. I can only expect that there has got to be something better on the other side of this for me because this cannot be as good as it gets for me. Not by a long shot!

This cannot be the beginning of my end either. I cannot imagine that it could be possible. I have had too few years granted to me– only 31– for God to take me any time soon. Though I don't know where life may lead me after this wild, unexpected, devastating, and challenging journey, I know that there are still way too many things that I want to do in this life. I have only begun reaching for the stars and chasing my dreams!

I want to find that one person that truly brings me all the happiness in the world...if even for a short time. I want to have my dad walk me down the aisle, as he has always dreamed of doing, and dance with him to Sweet Melissa by The Allman Brothers as the father/daughter dance. I want to see my parents grow old (sorry mom and dad) and take care of them as they have taken care of me. I want to see the world for myself instead of through pictures or through the television. I want to take my nieces shopping and spoil them like crazy. I want to see all three of them grow up to become independent, strong-minded, and good-hearted women. I want to see them go to their first prom and walk through their high school and college graduations, and I want to be around for when they get married and have children of their own.

I want to continue making memories with my family and friends. I want to keep looking for that next big adventure and hope that I have to white-knuckle it the whole ride (skydiving was not enough). I want to achieve great things in my career. I want to help at least one person (but more would be great) through their journey in the cancer world. I want to make it to the other side of this without having regretted anything and to become stronger and wiser for having gone through it...to see that silver lining. So, if after walking through the rain (the diagnosis, surgeries, chemo, radiation, continuous screening, etc.), I am provided with a second chance at life to do all the things I want to do, then I will have found my rainbow!!

Wednesday, May 23, 2007
Hey Doc, I will take $30.00 of premium!

I went in for my first "fill" with Dr. Gimbel, my plastic surgeon, today. It was rather uneventful and less frightening than what I thought it would be. They use a magnetic device to locate the port in my tissue expander, insert a needle, and begin to fill the foobies (fake boobies). Though I apparently have more feeling than most people do, it didn't really hurt. I couldn't feel the needle going in, but the sensation of being filled up was very odd. I couldn't help but giggle the entire time. I think this was much to my relief, as well as theirs, considering I'm usually in tears when I'm there. They finally got a taste of my twisted sense of humor and seemed to enjoy that side of me. We all laughed throughout my entire visit. I asked all the important questions like when I can resume my normal activities (kickboxing, Pilates, boxing, belly dancing, etc.). When can I ride rollercoasters? When can I go skydiving again? And when I can start dressing like a girl again?

It seems as though it will be much longer than what I had anticipated for most of the things I want to do, but I'm still allowed to bike and walk, and I can ride rollercoasters! Though I do have to say that just when I was feeling some relief from the pressure on my chest, it is now back. Driving is difficult, breathing is a challenge, and I fear the next time I have to sneeze! I feel like I'm carrying cannonballs on my chest. At least I'm prepared for battle, I guess.

We talked about the fact that I now have to undergo radiation and the implications of that. Dr. Gimbel shared that in speaking with, Dr. Ahrendt, my surgical oncologist, and Dr. Sushil Beriwal, the radiation oncologist, they all feel we can wait 12 weeks before starting the radiation to get me "filled" up and to complete the exchange (replacing the tissue expanders with the implants). Thus, I am on the "rapid expansion plan," which means I go in every week to get my fill; I will recover for several weeks, and then surgery again. They decided a fast track reconstruction option would be better in an attempt to avoid having to complete the operation of taking muscle tissue from my back (latissimus-flap procedure) and putting it where the radiation will be concentrated, though it is not a for sure thing. We will have to wait until after the radiation is completed to know if that will be the case.

I go back next Friday for my next fill and then I have an appointment with the medical oncologist on June 4th.

(5:30 am addendum: Being told that I might experience some discomfort and a bit of tightness was pretty much the understatement of the year! I hurt so bad that it feels like I had surgery all over again. UGH! I can't find a comfortable position to sleep in, so trying to sleep is pointless, not to mention painful.)

Thursday, May 31, 2007
Letting Go of a Dream

There was one dream that I chose to leave out of my "After the rain...the rainbow" entry, which is my dream to one day have children. When I was younger, I never wanted to have children, but in my mid-twenties, I changed my mind. I always wanted to have two children- twins- a boy and a girl. Yes, I realize this comes down to genetics, but a girl can dream! The names I have picked out for them are Trenton Kincaid and Ellie Mae. However, after thinking things through since my last conversation with Dr. Ahrendt, surgical oncologist, I have decided to let go of this dream. I'm not going to have children. This, by far, was a much harder decision to make than the bilateral mastectomy. Of all the things I hate most about being diagnosed with cancer, this is it!

I will never know the joy of giving another person(s) life, to hold that little person in my arms, and love him/her with all the depth of my heart. I will never know what it feels like to look at a child that carries so much of me within him/her and to see those aspects that he/she has inherited. I have always wondered what this world would be like with a little Melissa (or two) in it. Would he/she have my personality, my sense of humor, my eyes, my hair color, my sense of adventure, and the other attributes that make me ME? I will never get to experience the excitement and joy of his/her first word or step. I will not know how scary it is to send him/her to the babysitter, to kindergarten on the first day, or off to college. I will never get to experience the hope that I am doing all that I can do to shape him/her into becoming a good-hearted, well-rounded, level-headed, loving, and independent individual. I will never get to experience any of the things that I would by having my own child(ren).

Though all these things keep running through my head about what I will never experience, I can't help but think about how this decision has made my parents feel. I shared it with them this past weekend, and it broke my heart. I could see the look of devastation on my dad's face as I told him that he would never have a grandbaby from me. I can't imagine how it must feel for them to see me suffering through cancer. It must be hard for them not to know if I will be granted another day or if someone will ever love me enough for me, and that they will never have a piece of me left in this world should I not make it through to their end.

This decision was very personal and hard. I'm sure some may question why I would be so devastated and upset over a decision I'm consciously making, it's because it is not one that I should have ever been forced to make.

Tuesday, June 5, 2007
Pain, Pain, Go Away...and how about stay away!

I went in for another fill up at the BP (breast pumping) station on Friday. It went pretty much like the first one, so I wasn't all that concerned. I could feel that my chest was tight, as was to be expected, but the pain started much sooner than the last time. It was after only about an hour and a half that I started having pain. I left work an hour early (on my first and only day back) to come home and rest. By late Friday evening, I was in severe pain...much worse than the actual surgery. I was having muscle spasms that were enough to knock my ass to the ground. On top of that, my breathing was shallow, and my back was hurting. Nothing I took for the pain was even beginning to take the edge off. I suffered through until the morning and finally called Dr. Gimbel. He prescribed me 1500 mg of a muscle relaxer 4x a day. Thankfully, my friend Jill was able to go pick up the meds for me because I would never have been able to get them myself. Even as the meds control my muscle spasms, they can't contain my concern. My breathing is still shallow, my back still hurts, and my meds run out today.

I tried to think of a way to explain the pain that I'm in, and this was the only thing I could come up with: imagine wearing a corset about 2 sizes too small. It is incredibly tight and hard to move around in. Sitting, standing, and lying down are all now a challenge. Every move you make must be deliberate and well-thought-out. Getting in a good, deep breath is hard because you can't expand your lungs that much without it hurting. When you do try, you have to bend over to try to find the right angle to allow that to happen. And when you get it wrong, the pain shoots up into your lungs and rib cage. Your range of motion is limited, so you can't reach up in the air, twist to the side, or stretch. There is a relentless pain in your back from sleeping in an uncomfortable position for weeks on end. To top it all off, you have 2 cannonballs strapped to your chest! And if all that pain isn't already enough, you have to worry about someone making you laugh, or if you have to sneeze or cough. Oh, and did I forget to mention that you have to do PT exercises which consist of shrugging your shoulders, reaching up in the air, lying on your back and lifting your arms over your head? Also, you can't sleep at night because of all the pain. A simple activity such as the PT exercises takes you an hour and a half because you have to take a break to go lie down every so often. I hope that you will only ever have to imagine my pain and not actually experience this for yourself!

To give you additional perspective– Dr. Gimbel has me on a fast track. He is doing to me in two and a half months what is typically done over 6 months.

I go back in less than two weeks for what I'm hoping will be my last fill!!!

34

Tuesday, June 5, 2007
Chemotherapy

I met with my medical oncologist, Dr. Barry Lembersky, yesterday to find out if I need chemotherapy as part of my breast cancer treatment. To say my case is complex would be an understatement. I shouldn't have to make these heavy decisions. I am angry and overwhelmed. I don't know where to start...so here is a good place: The Oncotype DX test is conducted to determine the likelihood of cancer recurrence over ten years. The scores fall within the low-risk, intermediate, or high-risk range. My score falls within the intermediate range...the lovely gray area. Research studies have been conducted to determine the benefit of chemotherapy for those in both low- and high-risk ranges. Those who are at high-risk benefit from and need chemotherapy, whereas those at low-risk do not. Chemotherapy is typically recommended for those in the intermediate risk range; however, the benefits of it are unknown. Oh, joy!

Dr. Lembersky is leaving the decision for chemotherapy up to me. So, what does one in such a predicament do? Do I go through chemo to reduce the chance of recurrence (though it still may return) or do I choose not to have chemotherapy, as the real benefits are unknown?

Well, I guess some people would weigh the pros and cons of having to go through chemotherapy and make their decision based on that information. I, on the other hand, am giving up my choice as to whether or not I will have chemotherapy. I'm letting that decision be made by a computer...a coin toss if you will. You see, I am choosing to participate in a research study on the benefits of chemotherapy for those of us in the intermediate risk range. A random selection is made as to which of those participating in the research will receive only hormone therapy and which will receive hormone therapy plus chemotherapy. I had asked Dr. Lembersky the benefit of participating in the research study...not for me but for future breast cancer patients. I then told him that I would like to join in the research study, knowing I may have to go through chemotherapy and experience its side effects. He looked at me with astonishment and asked why. I said, "If I can do something today to help other breast cancer patients in the future, then so be it. I want to do something positive with this." He became teary-eyed and said that it has been a very long time since he has met a patient that has viewed her breast cancer experience with such altruism. I could only hope that everyone else would see it that way as well.

I have already been asked why I am choosing to participate in this study knowing full well I could make the conscious decision to avoid chemotherapy, and all that comes along with it. Let me first say that this is my decision, and I will do this. I will endure all that comes with the chemo should the computer randomly select my name for that treatment. Though it is a guarantee that I will lose my hair after the first treatment, and I may get sicker than a dog, the benefits of this research study outweigh all of those side effects. What I see down the road is a future breast cancer patient in a similar situation with better information regarding her treatment and being thankful for those of us who are here now participating in this study. I could only wish someone would have done this for me! And I can only respect and be thankful for all of those before me who have participated in other research studies that have improved upon the treatment for breast cancer.

I will end with this quote: "What lies behind us & what lies before us are small matters compared to what lies within us." ~Ralph Waldo Emerson

Sunday, June 10, 2007
The Reflection in the Mirror

I have heard a thousand times over how good I look considering all I have been through. While I appreciate hearing this and am thrilled that apparently, I am not what people expect a cancer patient to look like, I realize people associate looking good with feeling good and not being sick. One day, I sat looking at my reflection in the mirror wondering how it is that some people are missing the truth of the situation, the harsh reality of what I face every single day. Initially, when I see my reflection in the mirror, I see what everyone else sees- me, at face value– the façade. However, when I look deeper into my reflection, I see what most people either do not see or are truly afraid to see.

Reality is there is so much more behind those eyes and that smile than what anyone might be able to imagine. I see lines of worry on my face from something well beyond my years. I see a smile that isn't always genuine. Behind that smile is someone who feels isolated and alone...even when others are near. I see a smile that carries more sadness than true happiness. I see eyes filled with heartache, anger, frustration, and uncertainty, carrying deep, open wounds from the physical, emotional, and mental trauma that has been endured. I see eyes that have shed endless tears. I see eyes that carry the struggle of getting out of bed each morning and trying to live life despite being robbed of sleep each night. I see someone who has lost her life as she knew it; one who finds doing the smallest things is only an attempt to restore some normalcy into a life that has been turned entirely upside down. I see someone who has had to alter her view of what she thought this life would be and to let go of dreams that should have never been taken away. I see someone who wishes there were more to her life right now than just cancer. I see someone tired of the endless doctor's appointments and the daily consumption that cancer has on her life. I see someone who has endured a tremendous loss of life, friends, dreams, hopes, sleep, and even a loss of herself through all of this. The saddest part about looking at the reflection in the mirror is that after 31 years, I no longer recognize the person who is looking back at me.

If you ever see me face-to-face and don't look beyond the surface, you will be tricked every time into thinking that because I look good, I feel good.

Tuesday, June 12, 2007
Life Ain't Always Beautiful

As I sat here for most of the evening pondering life, people, and existence in general while shedding tears of anger, frustration, and sorrow, I realize that life is not beautiful. It is hard and sometimes it down-right sucks. There will be obstacles in life that we all must conquer...some more challenging than others, but the experience of having gone through it hopefully makes each of us stronger and wiser.

I sat with a great friend today and cried for some time over a horrific (to say the least) comment someone I don't even know made about my situation. She made a weak attempt at hurting my friend at my expense by telling him to "squeeze the one tit that she has left for me." To say I was angry would be an understatement. Though I do not know this girl, it took me back to a day when I was in my office crying with two secretaries in my office, Naomi and Cindy, asking them, "Who is going to love me now?" Though this girl will never know the impact of her statement, I realize some people are going to be heartless and callous about what I have been through for whatever reason. But I learned something valuable from this: though I may never understand why people do or say the things that they do or say, I can only see that it is a true reflection of their character- not mine. Despite how mean and hurtful someone might be about my situation; I am going to hold my head high and be proud that I am/will be a breast cancer survivor. I will carry the scars of my battle, knowing I faced it with dignity, courage, faith, hope, and love.

My friend and I talked about many other things as well, and I think the most profound topic for both of us was about wishes.

He said, "In this life, we are granted no wishes."

It's funny how we both agreed that if given a wish, we weren't sure the wish would be for me not to have cancer. Believe me, this isn't something I would have chosen, but I think that the experience has made me a different person in ways I may never know. Though every day continues to be a struggle, and there are still days that I put my head under the blankets for hours on end, and there are nights of endless crying, I'm not sure I would change who it is that I have or will become through this experience. It's not to say I don't like who it is that I see in the reflection in the mirror, it's that I am so different in so many different ways.

I think the lyrics from the country song, Life Ain't Always Beautiful by Gary Allan really hit the nail on the head with how I'm feeling right now: "Life ain't always beautiful. Sometimes it's just plain hard. Life can knock you down; it can break your heart. Life ain't always beautiful. You think you're on your way and it's just a dead-end road at the end of the day. But struggles make you stronger, and the changes make you wise. And happiness has its own way of taking its sweet time. No, life ain't always beautiful. Tears will fall sometimes. Life ain't always beautiful, but it's a beautiful ride.... I can dream, but life don't work that way. But the struggles make me stronger, and the changes make me wise. And happiness has its own way of taking its sweet time. No, life ain't always beautiful, but I know I'll be fine. Life ain't always beautiful, but it's a beautiful ride."

Sunday, June 17, 2007
Fill Up My Boobie

I went to see Dr. Gimbel, my plastic surgeon, for another fill up on Wednesday. As I always find it necessary to entertain him as well as the nurse (and myself), I sang to him, "Pump up the ta-tas" and "Fill me up Buttercup." There's nothing new to report on the BP station visit. Same old, same old. We confirmed the date for my next surgery, which will be next month (the day before my birthday– vomit. Happy birthday to me! I told the doc to be sure to bring gifts and a cake.) The outpatient surgery will be done at Magee.

I also went in for my range of motion test at Dr. Ahrendt's, surgical oncologist, office. I failed! That means I have to start physical therapy within the next few weeks. The only positive thing about that is the back massage I will be getting. I have to go back for a follow-up range of motion test on July 25th. The saddest part about the visit for me was not that I failed but that I was sitting in the waiting room and saw a young girl who was probably only 17 - 21 years old. I knew the reason she was there, as we are all there for the same reason. I can only guess that she was given the news that day, as I could hear her crying in the patient room. When Dr. Ahrendt walked out, she too was crying. I can't tell you how much I wanted to hug that girl, even though I didn't know her. I wanted to say to her that I'm sorry that she has to go through this and that I know how unfair it is. It broke my heart.

I meet with the medical oncologist, Dr. Lembersky, on Monday. I expect to find out if I have to go through chemotherapy then.

Monday, June 18, 2007
Chemotherapy Appointment #2

I went back to meet with Dr. Lembersky, medical oncologist, today regarding my decision to participate in the research study. I'm now officially pre-registered. They will be sending some of the tissue from my tumor, the results of my Oncotype DX testing, and the lab work I had done today for submission. Once all of that has been received and I am registered as a participant, the computer will determine whether I will receive hormone therapy alone or hormone therapy along with chemotherapy. The appointment was rather long but well worth it, in my opinion. I got stabbed three times with the needle before they were able to find a vein willing to cooperate. I have never had anyone try to take blood from the side of my wrist before, but I've had a lot of new things happen to me through this experience; chalk up another one.

I have such a hatred for needles, willingly sitting as they tried three times to take blood speaks volumes of my conviction to participate in this research study. During my third and final stabbing, I was taken down to the chemotherapy room. I had planned on visiting that area only if I would undergo chemo and it wasn't anything like what I had expected, I guess. I was relieved to see that they seem to try to accommodate the patients and make them as comfortable as possible. It touched my heart and brought tears to my eyes for reasons well beyond what most people can imagine unless of course, you have been through this. No one ever signs up for (or volunteers) to become a part of this sisterhood/brotherhood of cancer patients/survivors, but when you see another cancer patient/survivor who is fighting the fight and carries the wounds/scars of his/her battle, it inspires you and almost makes you proud to be a part of such an "elite" group.

Dr. Lembersky said he had thought about me many times over the past two weeks since we first met and shared that he feels my reasoning for participating in the research study is remarkable. Here again, I have to go back to my life goals of changing a life, making a difference, and touching a heart. As I said before, I have been provided the opportunity to do that in a way I can't even begin to grasp, but it is real, and I'm going to take advantage of it. He said again that it has been a long time since he has encountered a breast cancer patient who has dealt with her experience with such grace and desire to do something for someone else in the future, and for that, I told him that I am sorry. He reiterated the fact that I will lose my hair, but I assured him it was okay. I will accept whatever the computer decides for me. I may not like it, and there may be times that I question my sanity in doing this, but I know that in the end, I will have taken advantage of my opportunity to make a difference in someone else's life.

I should know next Monday if I have to endure the chemotherapy. If this is the case, it changes everything with the upcoming surgery and the radiation. The chain of events would be chemotherapy, surgery, and then radiation. I have an appointment scheduled for 8 am on July 3rd for my first chemotherapy appointment, just in case. This will result in my missing the second concert for which I had purchased a ticket. BOO!

If I am chosen to undergo chemo, I will receive four treatments approximately every three weeks. My medical team projects I will have my surgery to remove the tissue expanders and put in the implants sometime in late October or early November and then begin radiation a few weeks after that. So, when all is said and done, it won't be until at least January that I would be finished with these treatments.

I have my physical therapy evaluation tomorrow after work. I go back to the BP station and meet with the radiation oncologist on June 27th.

Wednesday, June 27, 2007
Moment of Truth

Everyone has been waiting to hear if I have been randomly selected to receive chemotherapy and believe me, I have been on the edge of my seat waiting for that phone call, as well. The moment of truth came today. I was selected to undergo chemotherapy, which will begin on July 9th. I'm still absorbing this information at the current moment, as it is a hard pill to swallow. I think it would have been hard even if I hadn't been selected but for different reasons, of course. I would be lying if I were to say that I'm not scared. I think this actually scares me more than having the mastectomy. I don't know what to expect, and the unknown has always been something I have struggled with.

I have so many thoughts going through my head about all of this, and there is a part of me that feels somewhat relieved that I have been selected because it is another precaution in an attempt to secure my future (though I do realize that nothing is a guarantee). But then there is a part of me that knows I will experience great sorrow over the loss of my hair. I also think about how people will react to me as they watch me go through this and how this will have an impact on them. The thing that outweighs everything is the thoughts about my nieces, other relatives, and even those I do not know who one day may walk down this same devastating path. Could I be so vain not to do all that I can now to change the future for someone else? And the answer to that is absolutely not. As I have told some others regarding the mastectomy (and I feel the same about this), I do not have to like it, I do not have to love it, and I do not have to embrace it. I will only accept it because I have life.

Plastic Surgeon visit
I went back for my final fill up with Dr. Gimbel, my plastic surgeon, today. He didn't give me a complete fill (60cc) because he felt that doing so would compromise my skin and the look of the foobies. He added 40cc of saline on both sides today and, so far, I have had only minor muscle spasms, which is nothing in comparison to what I had experienced previously. We canceled my surgery for July 16th. We anticipate I will undergo my surgery sometime in November. I'm not sure he sensed my sarcasm when I told him that my mom's birthday is November 1st if he wanted to go ahead and schedule it for that day, or maybe he didn't appreciate my humor. I won't see him again until after I have completed chemotherapy.

Radiation Oncologist
I finally met with my radiation oncologist today, Dr. Sushil Beriwal. Now that it has been determined I will be receiving chemotherapy, it was almost a waste of time, but it gave me comfort to finally meet him. He reiterated everything that Dr. Ahrendt, surgical oncologist, had discussed

with me– that the DCIS was too close to the margins (within a millimeter...eek) so as a precaution, radiation therapy was recommended. I will begin my treatment, which will last approximately five to six weeks of daily therapy Monday through Friday, following my surgery in November to replace the tissue expanders. He also discussed the possibility of having to undergo surgery to remove the tissue from my back to replace the tissue where the radiation will be concentrated. Statistically, the incidence of the radiation compromising the reconstruction is very high, which was very discouraging.

I will have to contact Dr. Beriwal following my last chemo treatment so that I can be scheduled for a CT Scan before beginning the radiation. As I was leaving the office, I was reminded of how young of a breast cancer patient I am when the nurse asked me if I was pregnant and I said, "NO!" She said that typically she does not have to ask that question because very rarely does she ever see someone of my age going through this. UGH!

Since I found out that I will be receiving the chemo, I picked up a knitted hat made by a local woman for my soon-to-be bald head. I love it because the tag says, "Each stitch is a prayer filled with love."

Though today was a stressful day and I have been on an emotional rollercoaster with all of this (again), I received the best thing today– my middle niece called me to say hello because she misses me. It took everything in me to not cry on the phone with her, but I told her how she made my day and brought the biggest smile to my face. She was so excited to talk to me and hear that I sounded well. What a great feeling it is to know that someone looks up to you so much and loves you unconditionally with all they have.

I came upon a quote today, and I didn't realize until I talked with my niece that the quote is actually a reflection of me. "I am strong, I am determined, and I am someone's hero." ~ Author Unknown

Monday, July 2, 2007
Enjoying Life

The past two weekends have been absolutely fantastic and have helped me to feel almost "normal" in this crazy mess that I call my life. Last weekend, I went to the Women of Faith conference in Cleveland with my friend Cathy. I felt so refreshed and renewed. It was very emotional and uplifting for me. I walked away with a lot, and a few things really stuck out. One of the speakers, Beth Moore, had driven home the message that we need to stop letting our WAS (past) and our IS TO COME (future) interfere with our IS (present). As I listened to her, I found that through my journey in the cancer world I have been able to let go of my regrets and grudges that are a part of my WAS and to release my fears and anxieties of my IS TO COME so I can focus only on my IS. Before all of this mess, I was as guilty as the next person in letting all of my previous baggage and my worries for the future interfere with the present. It is so true that we can't change our past and we can't predict our future, but we have such a hard time just living for today (the IS). I loved what another speaker, Patsy Clairmont, had said because it is so simple, yet so profound. She said, "Live Lively, Love Lavishly, and Forgive Frequently."

This weekend was very eventful. I went to Kennywood with my parents and a friend on Friday. It was my dad's work picnic day, which by the way, he works for Oncology Nursing Society (funny and ironic, I know). It was great to do something that I love with those that I love, but I have to say that some of the rides were not too kind to the foobies. I wore my "Cancer can take my ta-tas but it can't take my sexy" t-shirt. My friend wore his "I support ta-tas" t-shirt. It was amazing to me how many people had no clue what the t-shirts meant or why either one of us was wearing them. Of all the people that commented on our shirts, only one knew why we were wearing them. For me, it reconfirmed the fact that I need to do all that I can to increase everyone's awareness of this disease, especially in young women.

On Saturday, I went to a wedding in Erie for a dear, sweet friend, Julie. She and I worked together at Perseus House before I moved to Pittsburgh. It meant so much to me that I was able to share in her wedding day and see the beginning of her new life with her husband. Julie is such an amazing person. Though this was her special day, apparently, that was not the only thing that mattered. It brought me to tears and warmed my heart when she kissed and hugged me then told me, "Melissa, you made my day." It felt so good to know that my being there meant that much to her.

On Sunday, my friends from the Erie School District, the district I worked in before moving to Pittsburgh, organized a picnic at Presque Isle. It was a beautiful day to be out at the beach and surrounded by people who I know to love me. I can't thank everyone enough for coming. It meant the world to me. It was great to hang out and have people from different aspects of my life come together in one place. I walked down the beach with two of my friends after the picnic to take some pictures and enjoy nature's gifts. I have learned to enjoy the simple pleasures in life through all of this. I have never been one to enjoy the beach because I hated the feeling of the sand between my toes but, as I walked down the beach yesterday, I felt blessed that I'm still here to walk on the beach and feel the sand between my toes. It is a difficult thing to describe unless you have been there, but when you face your own mortality every single day, you take in all that you can and enjoy every moment of life because you realize tomorrow may not come. It's too bad it took this to learn that.

Today, I went to the Erie School District for lunch to visit with some of the folks who were not able to make it to the picnic. During lunch, my friend Bob Lansberry had shared a story about a woman's answering machine message that hit home with me after this weekend. It said, "I have made some changes in my life. If I do not return your call, you are not a part of that change." Though my weekend in Edinboro was terrific, I realized that I lost a large part of who I used to be pre-cancer. I learned that there are some of my "friends" who only liked the part of me that is no longer there, and I have been watching those friendships fade away as time passes. Through this journey, I have changed in so many different ways. I have learned so many things at the age of 31 that some people don't figure out in their entire lifetime. Like I told my friends today, sometimes I feel like I'm a 95-year-old mind trapped in the body of a 31-year-old. This may sound crazy, but I wouldn't trade the lessons I have learned.

Tuesday, July 3, 2007
CONFUSION!!!

I just received a phone call from Carol, who works at the Women's Cancer Research Center, to inform me that I have been randomized only to receive the hormone therapy- Tamoxifen. WHAT? I was so completely taken back by this since I had received the phone call from the secretary at my medical oncologist's office last week to reschedule my first round of chemotherapy. During my conversation with Mary, the secretary, she never communicated that I had been randomized to hormone therapy and not chemotherapy. After having gone through the emotional rollercoaster of thinking I would be receiving chemotherapy, I am now on a different emotional rollercoaster because I have not been selected. I'm completely beside myself and frustrated that a breakdown of communication could have occurred over something so important. I will express my concerns to Dr. Lembersky, my medical oncologist, since I had "pulled the plug" on the surgery for July 16th and the radiation therapy. Everything is back to where it was before, but unfortunately, I was already taken off Dr. Gimbel's surgery schedule on July 16th. I contacted his office to let him know that I will not be receiving chemotherapy and am waiting to hear back as to whether or not I can be put back on the schedule. Also, I spent an hour and a half of my time, as well as the representative from American Hairlines time, discussing my options for wigs and a hair prosthetic.

How frustrating!

Luckily, my surgery was rescheduled for July 16th (did I actually say luckily?). I have to make an appointment with my primary care physician, Dr. Andrews, to get the physical and go to Magee for blood work before I can have the surgery. I also spoke with Dr. Beriwal, my radiation oncologist, to let him know that I would not be receiving the chemotherapy. He was just as confused as I was about the whole situation. I will start my radiation therapy a month after my surgery.

Monday, July 9, 2007
How are You Doing?

Today I had an appointment with Dr. Lembersky, my medical oncologist. I initially saw the fellow working with him. The fellow is like the 9th or 10th person that I have seen since all of this started; I'm not sure how I keep all these people straight in my head, but somehow, I manage. He asked me to retell my story (clearly, he didn't read my chart) as if I haven't told it enough times. Truthfully, it doesn't get easier. I still have a hard time saying, "I'm 31, and I have breast cancer."

So once again, I go through finding the lump on February 20th up to the current day. He then asks me, "How are you doing?" Really, he should know better than to ask that question. He seemed stunned when I simply said, "I'm here." What more does anyone honestly expect? I'm not ecstatic; I'm not happy.

I'm sad; I'm nervous; I'm lacking sleep, and I hate just about every day because there isn't a day that goes by that this doesn't somehow consume a large portion of my life.

I brought up the miscommunication about the chemotherapy issue and was pretty clear about my feelings with that mix-up. The fellowship student checked my incisions, which are now completely healed, and then left. He returned with Dr. Lembersky and gave me a prescription for the Tamoxifen. The Tamoxifen is needed to decrease the level of estrogen in my body since my cancer cells are stimulated by estrogen. Dr. Lembersky checked my incisions as well. I think he finds humor in pressing on the center of the foobies and watching me jump right out of my skin when he does it. I think I would tolerate shock therapy much better than having someone press on the foobies like that. He talked with me about the side effects of the Tamoxifen and indicated that if I change my mind about chemotherapy, I need to let him know within the next few months. I assured him I am dedicated to this research study, and I will accept the hormone therapy alone.

He also brought up the removal of my ovaries again, which is a sensitive topic for me. I explained that I'm not ready to make that decision or to put my body through more trauma right now. I have called to get things started for the ovarian cancer screening, so I'm not ignoring it entirely.

After leaving my appointment, I had some lab work done for my surgery on Monday. As I sat waiting to be registered for outpatient services, I found myself crying but didn't know why. I think it's because I'm so overwhelmed with all of what is going on in my life and being the lone soldier in this battle day in and day out– I never get a break from it. The emotions and thoughts that swirl around in my head are more than what one person should have to deal with over a lifetime, let alone five months.

I filled my prescription for the Tamoxifen this evening. I never thought that looking at a pill bottle could make me cry, but I was wrong. It's very emotional when I think about the reason that I'm taking this medication. I have to take it for the next five years, so I will be 37 years old when my treatment for breast cancer is completely finished. The side effects are rather frightening. The thought of those, in addition to the side effects of the radiation, is enough to create much anxiety. The (potentially fatal) side effects of the Tamoxifen are cancer of the uterus, stroke, and blood clots in the legs and lungs. The side effects of the radiation are decreased red blood cell count (which will lower my ability to fight infection), damage to my lungs, and higher risk for other cancers. In addition, it is highly likely that the implant will rupture, which will require another surgery, and that the radiation will cause the existing tissue to shrink so I will need surgery to move the muscle from my back to my chest.

So how am I right now? I know I can't explain what my journey through the cancer world is like, but I'm hoping this gives some insight. As I listen to the lyrics of the song Stand by Rascal Flatts, it truly is an expression of how I feel and also how it is that I'm dealing with this—day in and day out:

"You feel like a candle in a hurricane. Just like a picture with a broken frame. Alone and helpless like you've lost your fight, but you'll be alright, you'll be alright. 'Cuz when push comes to shove, you taste what you're made of. You might bend 'til you break because it's all you can take. On your knees, you look up. Decide that you've have enough; you get mad, you get strong, wipe your hands, shake it off, then you stand. Life's like a novel with the end ripped out, the edge of a canyon with only one way down. Take what you're given before it's gone; start holding on, keep holding on. Every time you get up, get back in the race, one small piece of you falls back into place."

Monday, July 16, 2007
Surgery Day...Happy Birthday to the foobies.

No, I have not had my surgery yet. I'm trying to pass my time until my family (mom, dad, and Aunt Aggie) get here and take me to the hospital. I have to be there at 12:30 pm and surgery is scheduled for 2:30 pm. I suspect I will be in surgery for a few hours and then recovery for another few hours. I will probably be home sometime later this evening. I'm a bit nervous, but I think that is to be expected anytime you have to undergo surgery. I wasn't able to get much sleep last night. I was up and down several times throughout the night. One of my friends came over to hang out and ended up staying the night so that I wouldn't be alone (Thanks, Chuck!!).

Tuesday, July 17, 2007
Written by my BFF, Ken

Reconstructive/implant surgery went well for Melissa yesterday. The doctors actually took her a little earlier than her scheduled time. The surgery lasted about two hours, give or take. She was released from the hospital and spent the night at home under the watchful eye of her mother.

Melissa sounded a bit groggy last night as can be expected. She was, of course, her normal sarcastic but lovable self. Her biggest concern then was not being able to shower until Thursday so if you do try to venture over, take some air freshener or a clothespin!

She has a follow-up appointment later in the week (Friday) for a post-op visit with the doctors.

She is still quite tired and rather sore, but that won't slow down our "Sweet Melissa." She thanks everyone for their support, thoughts, and prayers. I am sure she will try to update again soon.

Thursday, July 19, 2007
July 16th- Surgery Day

I underwent my third surgery on Monday to have the tissue expanders removed and the silicone implants put in. My family (mom, dad, and Aunt Aggie) got to my apartment at 11:30 am, and we left for the hospital around 12 pm. I registered at Surgical Services at approximately 12:35 pm and was put on a "rush" status. When I asked why I was being rushed, the receptionist told me that Dr. Gimbel, my plastic surgeon, was ready to operate.

My family and I waited in the waiting room for approximately fifteen minutes before the nurse came to get me. I was taken into my pre-op room and prepped for surgery. The anesthesiologist came in to have me sign the consent forms. I had a hard time understanding him as he had a thick Asian accent. The nurse prepared me for the IV and was able to get it in on the first try. Dr. Gimbel came in while the IV was being put in and recognized my high level of anxiety. He drew on his canvas (AKA my chest) and then left. The nurse indicated that I would be ready for surgery in a few minutes, so I asked if I was going to be able to see my family before I went in for surgery. My parents and aunt were able to come back for only a few moments before they were ready to take me off to the operating room. They kissed me and told me that they loved me before leaving, and I started to cry. The nurse promised my family that they would take good care of me in the OR. I was given something through my IV to make me sleepy, but I was still coherent. The nurse that inserted my IV was not going to let me go until something was clarified with the anesthesiologist because he was reading my chart from the surgery on May 3rd. That made me nervous, but the nurse promised to clarify his misunderstanding before anything was done. I remember waiting to go into the OR, and the nurse was trying to scan my ID bracelet, but it wasn't working. I laughed and said, "You have to scan me to get your fuel perks."

Once I was taken into the OR, I remember seeing everyone getting things organized around me, and the Beatles were playing on the radio. Dr. Gimbel walked in, and I remember busting his chops about being a headbanger, as he was listening to heavy metal during his last operation. The nurse strapped my arms down and then put a gas mask over my face. I'm not sure what the anesthesiologist did, but it hurt like heck. I started moaning and groaning. The nurse instructed me to take several deep breaths. I took in two and then started having a hard time breathing. I started freaking out but couldn't move my arms to get the gas mask off. I was gasping for air, but she continued to hold it there on my face. That was the last thing I remember before waking up to see Dr. Ahrendt, my surgical oncologist, in the recovery room.

I'm not sure how long I was in recovery before they moved me to step down. The nurse kept trying to give me pain medication. After about the fourth time, I finally gave in to her request. After taking the meds, she moved me to step-down recovery. I was still fatigued and out of it. My mom came back first, and I only know that she kept tapping my hand to try to wake me up. My dad came back to be with me for a while, but I still wanted to sleep. After a bit, I felt like I was able to go to the bathroom– they make you void before they let you leave the hospital. The nurse stood there watching me; that was uncomfortable, to say the least. I sat for a little longer and then decided I could get dressed and ready to go. I was taken to the car via a wheelchair but was still so out of it that I was falling back to sleep on the way to the car. My dad and sister-in-law helped to get me into my apartment, which apparently was pretty funny. I was told that I looked like I was completely stoned. I had my sunglasses on and would walk only so far before I would stop and try to fall back to sleep. They got me into the apartment and on the chaise lounge. My aunt and sister-in-law went to fill my prescriptions.

I tried to eat but was only able to stomach four crackers with some peanut butter. The antibiotic makes me nauseous, and the painkillers make me tired. My mom stayed the night with me and then left the next day. I spent my birthday in my bed recovering from the surgery– it's not the most memorable birthday I have ever had, but it is one I won't soon forget! I'm finally able to shower today, but I'm nervous about unwrapping the "birthday presents" from Dr. Gimbel. I got used to what was there before, and now I have to get used to something else. I want to see, but at the same time, I don't. I think I might let Dr. Gimbel have the honor of unveiling the foobies tomorrow.

The next few weeks are filled with several appointments. I go for my post-op appointment tomorrow. I have my range of motion check on July 25th. On August 3rd, I have my first ovarian cancer screening appointment. August 7th is my CT scan. Ah, the life of a cancer patient.

Thursday, July 19, 2007
Unveiling= Emotional Trauma

Against my better judgment, I decided this evening that I would finally unveil the new foobies. At first, I could only bring myself to undo the Velcro front of my surgery bra and pull out the gauze. Immediately, I knew that I was not going to like what I was about to see. I had gotten used to seeing the tissue expanders and came to be okay with how they looked and felt. As I sat crying, I could feel that what is in there now is nothing like what I had expected. I touched here and there but still could not bring myself to walk into the bathroom and look. I sat on my couch and sobbed because I want "ME" back. I do not want this to be happening, and I cannot handle the emotional trauma of "losing me" all over again.

I knew that the foobies would not look and feel that same as my own breast tissue or even the tissue expanders, but I most certainly was not prepared to have them feel like water balloons and flattened pancakes. I know that though I may change on the outside, I am still me on the inside, but that does not make this any easier for me. It still destroys my self-esteem; just when I was starting to regain my self-confidence, I get knocked down again.

So after about an hour of sobbing on the couch, I figured I had made it this far so I might as well go and look. As I stood there in the mirror undoing the Velcro, I started crying all over again. I was devastated at what was before me. I HATE THEM!!

I continued to cry and repeatedly asked, "Why did he do this to me?" I sobbed the entire time I was in the shower and almost made myself throw up from crying so much. I tried to pull myself together when I got out of the shower, but no such luck. I lay on my bed and continued to cry for some time.

I have a thousand thoughts running through my head right now and am becoming angry with myself for feeling this way, angry that I have to deal with this, angry that I have been robbed of so much, and angry at life in general. I'm tired of everything that has come with this disease- my lack of self-esteem, my lack of sleep and energy, my inability to live my life without everything revolving around doctor appointments, treatments, and surgery, shedding countless tears, enduring the physical, emotional, and mental trauma, and dealing with this, day in and day out. It is wearing me down, and I am not sure how much more I have left.

Monday, July 23, 2007
Supporting Someone with Cancer Can Be Hard

I know it can be hard to support someone when you have no idea what that person is going through. Sometimes you don't know what to do or what to say, and you feel totally helpless. I want to be as gentle as possible with this so as not to offend anyone or to suggest that I'm not grateful for the support people have provided. But after much careful thought, I know that they would want me to be honest about this because I know that they genuinely care and want to help.

~Sometimes your positive energy has to be enough for the both of us. There are days when I don't have what it takes to get through the day, so I need you to pull me through.

~Forgive me if, in my fear of the unknown, I am difficult or unkind.

~Laugh with me and cry with me. I'm very good at hiding my tears to protect people from the pain that I suffer day in and day out, but sometimes I do need someone to wrap their arms around me and let me cry.

~Be honest with me.

~Be sensitive of my feelings. I am entitled to feel the way that I do, and despite all your efforts, there isn't much that you can say or do to change it.

~Please do not tell me that you understand what it is I'm going through when, in fact, you do not.

~Respect my need for independence. I don't like feeling fragile and helpless, so let me do what I can for myself.

~Remember that the scars on the outside are not as many as the scars on the inside, so even though I may look good on the outside, I'm still hurting tremendously on the inside.

~Touch me. Hold me. Hug me.

~Take the initiative. I'm not very good at asking anyone for anything.

~Tell me how you feel about what I'm going through. Engage in conversations with me about your thoughts and questions about my situation. I don't know what it is like to see someone of my age battling cancer. Share that with me.

~Please do not tell me what it is that you would do differently or how you think you would be if you were in my shoes. I'm genuinely doing the best I can, and there isn't a single person other than myself who knows what it takes for me to get up each morning and face the day.

~Listen to me.

~Do not minimize my situation. I need to be realistic about my circumstances and this disease. I do not consider myself to be lucky by any stretch of the imagination because I have stage IIA genetic cancer.

~Remember that it is okay to say nothing at all.

Sunday, July 29, 2007
Post-Surgery Follow-Up

Friday, July 20th, I went to see Dr. Gimbel so he could check my incisions. I had made good progress by making it through my last few appointments without shedding a tear, but unfortunately, I didn't get any further than the waiting room on this visit. The floodgates opened when his nurse, Judy, asked me if I was okay. She can read me like a book and knew there was something wrong. She sat hugging me as I sobbed about how much I hate the implants and how I want them fixed. When I saw Dr. Gimbel, he said he is pleased with the outcome of the surgery. I couldn't even begin to tell him how devastated I am without sobbing. I sat there with tears falling down my face while Judy explained to him why I'm not happy with the outcome. He explained to me that he had to drop down the size of the implant because my skin would not be able to tolerate the larger of the two implants; it would have been too tight. Dr. Gimbel said to give it some time. If I'm still not happy with it, then he will fix it in a year. I made an appointment to see him again on August 22nd and then left his office feeling no better than what I had when I walked through the door. I was barely able to control my crying enough to drive myself home, but I managed to get back safely.

I sat out on my back patio, crying and rocking back and forth in a chair, for about four hours. I didn't want to talk to anyone or see anyone. I think that this day was probably the closest I had ever gotten to actually "shutting down" during all of this. I had built up a lot of anger and frustration from the day before with no real, good outlet to release it (a punching bag would have been great). My friend found me on my back patio and talked to me for a few minutes. I could see the pain in his eyes as he stood there, looking at me curled up in a ball rocking on this chair with tears in my eyes and heartache in my voice. I forced myself to get dinner and then tried to get some sleep, but I was still too angry and devastated to let my body and mind rest.

On July 25th, I went in for my range of motion test at my surgical oncologist's office. No one ever did check to see if I had regained my range of motion. They were more concerned with the fact that I was so emotional over the outcome of the reconstruction. I talked to two nurses before Dr. Ahrendt was able to see me. I wasn't on her schedule for the day and didn't want to bother her with this because I know that she is busy and there truthfully isn't anything that she can do about it. All agree that the most important thing is for me to be comfortable with myself. Dr. Ahrendt looked at the reconstruction and said that it indeed was the "best" that they could realistically do in making them look like my own breasts in terms of shape and feel. She listened as I explained my concerns, which are well beyond the look, feel, shape, and size. She reassured me that I made the best decision that I could have based on the information that I had, especially given the fact that I'm a genetic carrier. I agreed and explained that I wouldn't undo that decision, but I very much feel that I need to be comfortable in my own skin. I don't like looking at myself, I don't like showering, and I hate getting dressed. I can't wear some of my clothes because of how self-conscious I am about the foobies. One of the reasons I respect Dr. Ahrendt is because she gives it to me straight.

She said, "As you know we have no cure for cancer. I wish that we did. I can't offer you any guarantees for anything with this. All I can give you is a hug. You truly have been dealt a very unlucky hand." I thanked her for her honesty and hugged her. I see her again next May for my annual check-up.

It hasn't gotten any easier to look in the mirror at myself or to accept the changes, but I won't let that get in my way of facing the world every day. There are days when I need to be by myself to sort through my thoughts and feelings. I'm okay with being pissed off and crying for a day or two every so often as long as I get back up and continue on with my battle. I know a lot of people get worried about me sometimes when this happens, but I think this will help. On the way home from the hospital on July 16, a song came on the radio that I like and in my doped up and physically incapacitated state, I said to my dad, "I'm dancing on the inside." Trust me, even if I'm physically unable to get up and "dance" through this thing called life every so often, know that I'm still dancing on the inside. No matter how hard things may get, I will never, ever surrender my spirit to this disease. One day, it may be all that I have left.

Through living, I have learned to die. And through dying, I have learned to live. And, I'm going to LIVE STRONG.

Sunday, August 5, 2007
Ovarian Cancer Screening

On Friday, August 3rd, I went for my first ovarian cancer screening. The appointment took approximately two and a half hours, so I was utterly exhausted by the end of it. The ultrasound was completed first. The technician was good about explaining what I was looking at on the screen because I honestly had no idea; it all looks like a bunch of black and white scribbles to me. She indicated that everything looked typical for the most part except for something of slight "suspicion" on my left ovary, but she wasn't concerned. Hmm...

I asked her when ovarian cancer is detectable, and she said not until a mass has formed. Oh, goody, that's comforting. I was sent back to a patient room after the ultrasound and waited to be seen by the geneticist despite my giving them the results of the genetic testing. I sat for what seemed like forever before Darcy Thull, the geneticist I worked with at Magee, came in to see me. It was more like a therapy session than anything else, but it was okay because she is going to try to make a connection with me and some other breast cancer patients in a similar situation. I also asked her to give my name and number to any young breast cancer patients that would like someone to talk with.

I waited about forty-five minutes before Dr. Kristen Zorn, and her team met with me. I sat there and listened intently despite already having known most of what she communicated. I already know I'm at high risk for ovarian cancer because of the genetic mutation, I know that ovarian cancer cannot be detected in the early stages, and I'm aware that the rest of my womanhood is wanted by the time I'm 35 years old. I listened less intently as she explained the surgical procedure for removing the uterus, ovaries, and fallopian tubes...not out of ignorance, but out of denial. It is beyond my comprehension that I have to give up all of my womanhood to save my life as a result of my own self-destructive genetic makeup. *vomit*.

They suggested I start planning a family now, to which I responded, "Well, that is kind of hard to do considering my current situation: Single."

Maybe I should put an ad in the paper that says, "Cancer patient with genetic mutation seeking single male for baby-making. Needs to be done ASAP. Ovaries have to be removed by age 35. No dating required."

Dr. Zorn recommended that I go through the ovarian cancer screening process once a year. She reviewed a clinical research study currently being conducted with BRCA1 and 2 carriers, which I opted to participate in. As a result, I had to have four tubes of blood drawn, three for the study and one for the CA-125 (which is an ineffective blood test used to help identify ovarian cancer as it can indicate a false positive).

Though I didn't go into this with Dr. Zorn, I feel many things go into the decision regarding childbearing that I'm not sure it is fair I make them on my own. It is possible to make gene selection through in-vitro fertilization so a child could be "created" without the genetic mutation. However, on the other side of that is the estrogen factor– pregnancy increases estrogen levels, and estrogen stimulates my cancer cells. So, what cost would I have to pay to have a child? And taking Tamoxifen until I'm 37 puts me two years beyond my "deadline" before I can even consider children. BLAH!! I know where I stand on the issue, but I whole-heartedly believe this is something that should be discussed with a partner. On top of all of that, dating isn't even a priority of mine right now. I don't have time to focus on someone else's needs. It's all about me at the moment.

Sometimes I feel like I'm stuck between reality and my own worst nightmare and am constantly bouncing back and forth from one to the other. I'm not sure how I can explain this, but there are days when I'm upbeat and living life, and then there are days when I can't break away from all of the terrorizing thoughts and have a hard time with everything. I try to keep the two separate in hopes of maintaining some level of normalcy in a world turned upside down, but it is difficult when my reality IS my own worst nightmare come true.

My CT scan is on Tuesday and radiation begins the following week.

Tuesday, August 7, 2007
CT Scan

I went for my CT scan today to prepare for my radiation therapy, which will begin on August 20th. I first met with a nurse, Dr. Beriwal, Dr. Marsha Haley, and an intern. Dr. Haley and Dr. Beriwal marked the area where the CT scan needed to be conducted, which is also the area where the radiation will be concentrated. The plan is to treat a more substantial area (vertically from about three inches below my collarbone down to about one and a half inches from the bottom of my rib cage and horizontally from my sternum over to the side of my rib cage) for five weeks and then a localized area during the sixth week. I asked both Dr. Beriwal and Dr. Haley if the cancer was within only 1mm of the margin and Dr. Ahrendt went in as far as she could, is there a possibility that there is more cancer and got an answer from the both of them that didn't satisfy the question. I was only told that if there is any residual microscopic cancer left, theoretically, the radiation will destroy it. I guess I didn't ask my question correctly because I just wanted to know if it were possible for cancer to have spread my trunk considering that they found cancer cells in my abdominal wall during my mastectomy.

As I was being prepped, I asked the nurse about a thousand questions. To my dissatisfaction, I'm not allowed to shave or wear deodorant for six weeks. Oh yeah, I'm going to be hairy and smelly...how sexy is that?? I'm thinking of changing my newspaper ad to say, "Hairy and smelly cancer patient with genetic mutation seeking single male for baby-making." Surely that will make them all come running!

She seemed to enjoy my humor when I told her that it is a good thing that I don't have a hot and heavy date planned for this weekend for which I would be taking my clothes off. We both agreed that the big purple Xs around my boob might be a good icebreaker though.

After I was prepped for the CT scan, I was sent over to the CT/MRI center. I waited for about 45 minutes before being taken back. I didn't have to consume any contrast or have an IV put in like some of the other folks did, which was fine by me. It took approximately ten minutes and was less intimidating than most of the things I have experienced through this. When I was finished, the nurse put a few pieces of tape on the marks that cannot be removed so I have to be careful when I'm showering and I can't sweat, which doesn't work for me since I've decided to resume my workout routine. I wonder what will happen if the marks do disappear–will I get detention? Worse yet, will I not get radiation? Hmm...this may be something to consider. Anyway, I go back later next week for my pre-radiation appointment to discuss proper care of the skin, since they are pretty much going to be burning the hell out of me. But hey, it will be the only suntan I get this summer.

I had a message on my answering machine from the High-Risk Ovarian Cancer Center today. The lady said that it was nothing urgent, but she needed to talk to me about my blood work. Um...newsflash...just the fact that she called sends up red flags that the CA-125 may have come back positive. And though I do know that the test can indicate false positives, it does not sit well with me since I know I'm genetically predisposed to developing ovarian cancer. I called back, but she was gone for the day. I will call again tomorrow, as I'm slightly on edge.

Sunday, August 19, 2007
Radiation...Coming Soon

Well, tomorrow is my first radiation treatment. I'm a little nervous, because I'm not sure what to expect and I think the unknown is always somewhat intimidating.

I went last Thursday (August 16th) for a pre-radiation appointment. It took about a half-hour for the technician to take some x-rays and a photo of my mug and to line up the fields for the radiation. I was fine at first but started to become emotional partway through the process. I'm not sure what scared me about it. Realistically, it was one of the least invasive things I have experienced through all of this, but it still freaked me out. My purple Xs and stickers were removed but only to have new, bigger ones put on me. Apparently, I will be tattooed after the first week of radiation.

After all of the technical aspects of the appointment were completed, I sat down with the nurse to review how to care for the irradiated area. I was already pretty well-prepared (had the deodorant without aluminum, cotton bras, and dove soap) but still need to find some clear aloe vera gel. I have looked everywhere for it but cannot find any that doesn't have something added to it. The nurse reviewed some of the side effects of the radiation with me. I will burn where the radiation is concentrated, I may become fatigued (my medication already does this, but I still can't sleep), and my immune system may not be as strong. And of course, I already knew about the other "exciting" effects of radiation– may cause other cancers, may rupture my implant and may result in my having another surgery.

I go for radiation at 8:30 am, five days per week for about six weeks. I see Dr. Beriwal at the beginning of every week. I will miss two days of radiation that will need to be made up at the end of the six weeks, as I am going to Florida for a few days at the end of this month. Finally, something for ME!! Oh, how sexy am I going to be in my bikini with four big purple Xs on me? Now ask me how much I care!

I have made it through my first month of the Tamoxifen. Only fifty-nine more months to go! But hey, who is counting?

Tuesday, August 21, 2007
Radiation- Treatment #1

I went in for my first radiation treatment yesterday. The appointment took about 35 minutes. The actual "zapping" only takes a few minutes. They "zapped" me for approximately twenty-five seconds from two different angles. The radiation machine and the noise kind of freak me out. I have an automatic flight response when the machine is rotating around me– I want to jump off the gurney and run. But I didn't. I sucked it up and took it like a champ (or so I would like to think). I'm not sure which was worse though, the machine and the noise, or the assisting nurse poking me in the side. As I was being prepped, she put a protective covering over my scar and poked me in the area just below my right armpit. I don't know how to describe the feeling that I have there; when she poked me, I about jumped right out of my skin...literally. It went through my whole body, and my feet actually came up off of the table. It was as bad as the medical oncologist poking me in the center of the foobies. It's cruel!

I think I'm going to wear a sash from now on that says "Caution, Under Construction." That might prevent the doctors from poking and the bear hugs that some people like to give.

Today was radiation treatment number two, but who is counting? Oh, wait, yes, that would be me! It was relatively quick (about fifteen minutes), and they were more than willing to oblige when I asked them not to poke me. I had that flight response again, though, so I'm going to purchase an iPod this weekend so that maybe it will help me to relax. I close my eyes, but it doesn't do much for me.

I have my radiation appointment tomorrow, then I see the plastic surgeon right after.

Wednesday, August 22, 2007
Radiation and Plastic Surgeon Visit

Radiation treatment number three was today– only twenty-seven more to go. Ugh…it seems never-ending. The appointment took a little longer today because the techs were running behind with the patient before me. I got permission to bring an iPod to listen to so I can focus on something other than the machine and the noise. I'm starting to notice some slight changes in the area being treated; the skin is getting pink, and I am sensitive to the touch.

Following my radiation appointment, I went to see my plastic surgeon, Dr. Gimbel. I had been dreading this appointment because of how difficult the last one was for me. Dr. Gimbel and I talked about how upset I was during my previous visit; I reassured him that my opinion of the implants has not changed. I still hate looking at myself in the mirror. I tried to explain to him that it isn't just about size, but I became frustrated and simply told him that as a man, he will never understand what I'm going through. By the time I am 35 years old, I will have been stripped of all the things that I believe make me a woman, not to mention already having my hopes and dreams taken away. Thus, it is crucial for me to feel an acceptable level of comfort with my body. I need to be comfortable with myself before I can let someone close enough with hopes that he will be comfortable with me as well. I can't even begin to imagine in my head how that scenario is going to play out. It is very frightening for me to imagine myself allowing someone to see what only I see (and hate).

We talked about the recreation of a nipple and tattooing of the areola. Dr. Gimbel feels that this can be done about six months post-radiation. I asked him if when the nipples are recreated, would it look like I'm smuggling Tic-Tacs? His expression was priceless, and he responded that it would. So, to follow up with that, I asked him what the real function of the nipple is and, of course, he completely missed my point because he started talking about breastfeeding. Um…yeah, that would be interesting in my case. So, I clarified by telling him that I couldn't come up with a good use for the recreated nipples other than the possibility of hanging Christmas decorations from them. And I wonder why he looks at me like I'm completely out there. Anyway, he was adamant about my not having the surgery to switch the implants for another year, which is very much to my dismay.

He repeatedly said, "If that is the choice you make," when discussing that surgery. Newsflash– none of this was by my choosing. I do not remember saying, "I would like to have an order of genetic breast cancer with the possibility of ovarian cancer on the side, and I would like to top them with a bilateral mastectomy and removal of my ovaries." I forgot to ask for the cherry on top, apparently.

Dr. Gimbel explained what I should be looking for during radiation concerning changes in the implant/skin, which may result in undergo another surgery (tightness, change in the symmetry, and hardening of the implant). He took some photos and then told me how great he thinks they look. Before I could even say it, he said, "But I know it doesn't matter what I think." Ding, ding, ding! He wants to see me in six months post-radiation (March/April) unless I notice any of the changes he mentioned.

As I was leaving, his nurse asked me if I was okay because I clearly had "disheartened" etched all over my face. I said I would be fine and left the office, but before I could even get outside, I started crying. I cried all the way to school and through most of the morning. I'm looking for a small glimmer of hope that there is a light at the end of the tunnel. I just can't see it right now, and that is frustrating...twenty-seven radiation treatments, six months to see the plastic surgeon again, one year before I can have the other surgery, fifty-nine months of Tamoxifen left...blah, blah, blah. It is hard to get on with living my life when I have the "Big C" looming over my head. I try; I honestly do, but sometimes it catches up to me and pulls me back down.

Take the most horrific thing you have ever endured in your life, magnify it by a thousand, and imagine living through it day after day with no end in sight. This is how I feel. I take it one day at a time, but when that one day at a time is a continuous repetition of the hell the day before, it wears me down. Though cancer may have broken my body, and I swear to protect my spirit and my soul, I would be lying if I said that it doesn't wear them thin. I realize I'm having significant body image issues that need to be dealt with and no matter how many times people tell me how "great" I look, I can't see beyond the brokenness.

Tuesday, August 28, 2007
Daddy's Little Girl

I was at my Aunt Darlene's (my mom's sister) wedding this weekend. My Uncle George, brother of my biological father, was even in attendance. My mom had spoken with him, and he told her he would like for me to go see him. My first reaction was not necessarily a positive one, as I have had nothing to do with most of the paternal side of my family for many years. After I thought about it, I realized there was a time, a lifetime ago, that this man was involved in my life, so I went over and spoke with him briefly. I wasn't expecting to be brought to tears during my conversation with him.

Uncle George started talking about my grandfather, whom I absolutely adored. We talked about my last visit with him in the hospital before his passing. Then he said the unthinkable...he referred to my biological father as "your dad." I quickly interjected and said, "Just so you know, when you or anyone else says 'your dad,' you are referencing the only father I have ever had in this life, and he happens to be standing back there." My Uncle George went on to say how he couldn't believe that my biological father hasn't made contact with me. I very passionately told him there is absolutely NO reason for that man (and I use that term loosely) to ever call me...most certainly not now, after 32 years of missed opportunities. Uncle George apologized and recognized that it is no one's fault but his own that I do not wish to speak to him. I have had many arguments with many family members over the years because I have refused to call him my "father" or "dad." They would become angry with me, but I know who my father is and have known who my father is my entire life.

I ended my conversation with Uncle George and requested the DJ play the song that MY DAD says reminds him of me– My Little Girl by Tim McGraw. I ran across the hall to him and made him stop bartending to come and dance with me. As we danced, I think everyone was watching us, but for those few minutes, it felt like we were the only two in the room. We listened to the words for some time when he looked at me and said, "You know, this song is so true." At that point, both our eyes welled up with tears, and I'm sure others did, too. There is a part of the song that says, "One day some boy's going to come along and ask me for your hand. But I won't say yes to him unless I know that he is the half that makes you whole, he has a poet's soul and the heart of a man's man. And I know he will say that he's in love, but between you and me, he won't be good enough."

I looked at him and said, "One day, dad, one day." He hugged me tighter, knowing the pain in my heart and my fear that I'm the one who won't be good enough. We danced the rest of the song without saying much, but I had a thousand memories of this man who holds me so close to his heart running through my head– a man who 30-some years ago had no obligation to take on the responsibility of raising two children who were left behind by a coward. A man who looks at me not as the child of another man, but as a child of his own creation. A man, who no matter the circumstances, will always see me as his little girl.

This is part of a poem written by a father (Steve Kandel) whose daughter, Sari, lost her battle with breast cancer. I thought it may be a reflection of how my parents feel.

> I awake at 3:00 with a start
> with an ache in my heart
> maybe this heaviness will go if I write
> organize my thoughts...nothing trite
> I still see you in my mind's eye
> sitting beautifully erect as you try
> to keep our bearings before they start
> you know we will, soon, be apart
> absent your eyebrows, lashes, and hair
> your radiance and bravery so striking I stare
> you return my direct gaze
> perhaps knowing my thoughts through the haze?
> but then I see a twinkle in your eyes,
> yes, Daddy, I know you love me, and I you, no surprise
> the nurse questioning you
> when will she be through?
> but she turns to me and says "I will take good care of your daughter"
> and I know in my heart she will
> the hours anxiously waiting and getting the good news
> then magically seeing you in recovery
> when they adjust your bed I see the shock as your breath is taken away
> a pain so intense, even with morphine, you cannot speak...nothing to say
> except a gasp, the panic I see in your eyes
> my heart breaks a little then
> I know it will pass
> but seeing my child, suffering so, disturbs me to my core
> no parent wants to see a daughter go through this
> but it is a necessary journey, life-saving journey
> you have intelligently embraced.
>
> Love ya Dad!

Thursday, September 6, 2007
Stepping Outside of the Box

For the past five months, I have been living inside of this little box...surrounded on all four sides by nothing other than everything cancer. This past weekend, I went to Palm Beach, Florida with my friends Naomi and Heidi and met up with my friend Amy, who recently moved from Edinboro to Boynton Beach.

This weekend was the first time I allowed myself to venture outside of the cancer box and just be Melissa– not Melissa, the breast cancer patient.

I wouldn't say that I threw caution into the wind, but I would definitely say that I was much more carefree during those four days than what I have been over the past five months. I was very much living in the moment the entire time I was down there, and I wasn't as concerned as I typically am about the things that I should or shouldn't be doing as a good little cancer patient. I always feel like I'm trapped by cancer, but this weekend, I almost felt like my life was normal again. Cancer wasn't at the forefront of all of my thoughts; not to say that I didn't talk about it or that I didn't think about it at all, but it most certainly didn't consume my thoughts as it usually does. My first thought when waking up in the morning was not to put my head under the blankets in hopes that it would all go away. It felt so good to do something for me finally.

While there, I met a man that I had a mutual attraction to and actually allowed myself to flirt with, talk to, and dance with. My comfort in doing that was very much driven by the fact that I knew there was no chance in hell that my interactions with this man would lead to anything intimate where I would need to tell him about my situation. We had so much fun together, and it felt good that he only knew me as Melissa. Through email, I have since shared with him the fact that I have breast cancer not knowing what his response would be– fearing the worst. To my satisfaction, his reaction was not a negative one, and he actually gave me his phone number because he said he would love to talk to me *smiling*. Though I have no expectations of anything with this guy, it makes me feel a little better about myself. It also made me feel good when another guy that was with our group told me that, "Cancer or no cancer, you are truly an amazing person and the best part about the night was the fact that you looked like you were having more fun than anyone of us." It was very much the break that I needed from all of this, and though I knew my trip would quickly come to an end, I enjoyed every single moment while I could.

I resumed my foobie zapping (radiation) on Tuesday, which is now taking a significant toll on my body. It has me completely fatigued and is making me nauseous about a half-hour after I receive the treatment. I feel like someone put a vacuum in my mouth and sucked all of the life out of me, and I want to vomit all over the place (pleasant thought, I know). I don't have any energy to do anything at all...I just don't want to move. It takes everything in me to do the smallest tasks, but I keep pushing forward, slowly but surely. Even though I'm exhausted enough to actually go back to sleep after my ritual 3 a.m. waking, sleeping doesn't make the fatigue go away, and it keeps getting progressively harder every day. This is so much fun...eighteen more treatments to go!!

Tuesday, September 11, 2007
Lonely Soul

Under most circumstances, I'm usually reasonably content with being on my own. I have always enjoyed the freedom of doing things when I want and how I want without having to take someone else's feelings and wants into consideration. I have always been, as someone once described me, "freakishly" independent. Up until the day that my life changed forever, I relied on very few people for very few things. The only person that I ever expected to pull through for me when I needed something was, well, me. I'm not sure if it was a blessing or a curse, but it is the reality of the way I had been most of my life. I think it was a way of protecting myself from ever being let down by anyone. If you have no expectations from anyone, how can anyone ever let you down?

Well, I have been sitting here for most of the evening wondering how things would be different if I had someone to walk beside me through all aspects of this journey. I have some people that come pretty close in that regard; they do the best they can with what is going on in their own lives, but there is a lot of time that I spend alone– just me and my cancer. Those are the moments when I wish I could reach out to someone and have him wrap his arms around me. I find that I want someone to protect me from all the ills in this world because I feel like I haven't done a good job of that on my own. I want someone to wipe away all the tears that I shed when I'm by myself. I want someone to hold me through the night when I can't sleep from all the terrorizing thoughts swirling around in my head. I want someone to share my thoughts with– someone who won't tell me not to think a certain way or to say certain things because he can't face the reality of what life has handed me. I want someone who isn't focused on fixing all of what is broken but rather, embracing me in all of my brokenness. I wish for one moment there were someone here to help carry some of the burden I have weighing on my shoulders, day in and day out. If I could only have but one wish...

Wednesday, September 12, 2007
Battle

I find a lot of comfort through music in dealing with my cancer journey. I recently "met" a guy online who had an older brother die from cancer at the age of 31. Keith has had a tremendous impact on my life and my battle against cancer. He has been a blessing that came out of nowhere. He introduced me to this song by Colbie Caillat that I find to be an accurate reflection of my feelings and thoughts about my situation. It makes me think about so many things– how I felt so carefree and invincible pre-diagnosis, the day I was diagnosed, all the decisions I have had to make, how I have had to put all my faith in my doctors to try to save my life, how someone that has had nothing to do with me my entire life has shattered my world as I knew it, how cheated I feel by life, and how I continue to be the lone soldier in this battle every single day.

Anyway, here are the lyrics, but if you can get your hands on the actual song, you will love it.

> You thought we'd be fine. All these years gone by. Now you're asking me to listen while they tell me about everything. No lies, we're losing time. 'Cuz this is a battle and it's your final last call. It was a trial, you made a mistake, we know. Why aren't you sorry, why aren't you sorry, why? This can be better, you used to be happy...try.

> You've got them on your side. They won't change their minds. Now it's over and I'm feeling like I missed out on everything. I just hope it's worth the fight. 'Cuz this is a battle and it's your final last call (why'd you have to let it go). It was a trial, you made a mistake, we know (can't you see you've hurt me so). Why aren't you sorry, why aren't you sorry, why? Things can be better; you can be happy...try.

> 'Cuz this is a battle and it's your final last call. It was a trial, you made a mistake, we know (can't you see you've hurt me so). Why aren't you sorry, why aren't you sorry, why? This can be better; we can be happy if we try.

> 'Cuz this is a battle and it's your final last call.

Thursday, September 13, 2007
Radiation Oncology Reports

This week made three weeks of radiation on Tuesday. I'm more than half-way through now! Woo Hoo! When I went in on Monday, the techs indicated that more films needed to be taken. I was surprised because we did that on Friday last week. So, being the curious being that I am, I asked, "Why?"

I was told that some "changes" needed to be made. Okay, explain. I was then told that some "adjustments" needed to be made. I wanted to know if they were adjusting to treat more or less of the breast area. Finally, it was conveyed that the radiation oncologist wants an additional 3mm of my lung treated. Hold on; wait a minute! My lung? I have breast cancer, not lung cancer, right? I inquired further and was told that to treat all of my breast tissue, they had to treat the lung as well. Um...I have NO breast tissue. The tech tried to make light of the situation by telling me that 3mm was "nothing really." Well, sure it is nothing when it isn't YOUR lung and you are protected from the radiation by a huge lead door! This did not sit very well with me, so on Tuesday, I asked for my records, which were given to me on Wednesday. They seemed a bit uptight when I asked for the information. I wanted all of my lab results, but they said I would have to go through medical records for that information.

My bedtime reading last night consisted of my radiation oncology consultation report. I'm not sure if it is a blessing or a curse that I now understand cancer terminology. My heart dropped as I read through the report. I wanted to crawl up into a ball and put my head under the blankets to shut the world out in hopes of making it all stop for a moment. The unfortunate thing is that it never stops, not even for just a moment. In reading the report, the reality of how close my cancer was to both my pectoralis muscle and abdominal wall hit me in the face...only to be dropped on my ass by reading that, "In her case, in view of close or positive margins, she is at high risk for recurrence."

How much can one person truly take? I whole-heartedly believe that God only gives you what you are strong enough to handle but damn, give me a break already. I'm hardly made of steel, and I can only be strong for so long before I come crashing down. Though I have been a realist about my situation when most of my family and friends want to see it through rose-colored glasses, it was hard to see it on paper. It still breaks my heart that here I am, 32 years old and staring death straight in the face *flipping off the grim reaper*.

When I think of what I should be doing at this age, it is hardly this. I should be having the time of my life right now– sitting on top of the world, figuring out what I want in life, chasing my dreams, and reaching for the stars. Instead, I'm trying to have the time of my life because I have no idea how much life I actually have left.

There is a song called Fall by Clay Walker that is an accurate expression of how I feel about my always having to be so strong and my wanting someone to wrap his arms around me to protect me from the world.

"Oh look there you go again. Putting on that smile again, even though I know you've had a bad day. Doing this and doing that, always putting yourself last. A whole lot of give and not enough take. But you can only be strong so long before you break, so fall, go on and fall apart. Fall into these arms of mine. I'll catch you every time you fall, go on and lose it all. Every doubt, every fear, every worry, every tear I'm right here. Baby fall.

Forget about the world tonight, all that's wrong and all that's right. Lay your head on my shoulder and let it fade away. And if you want to let go, baby, it's okay. Fall, go on and fall apart. Fall into these arms of mine, I'll catch you every time you fall. Go on and lose it all. Every doubt, every fear, every worry, every tear I'm right here. Baby fall.

Hold on, hold on, hold on to me. Fall, go on and fall apart. Fall into these arms of mine, and I'll catch you every time you fall. Go on and lose it all. Every doubt, every fear, every worry, every tear. I'm right here. Baby fall."

Tuesday, September 25, 2007
Radiation Update

Well, I'm down to my last five treatments of radiation!! Woo Hoo!! I went in today for my final treatment to the entire breast area. The next five treatments will be boosts to the tumor bed. New films and pictures were taken, and Dr. Beriwal, radiation oncologist, drew a circle about the size of my fist on my chest. It's like tic-tac-toe...x's and o's. He is a little concerned about the scar, as it is inflamed and looking pretty nasty despite my consistently using the aloe vera. In addition to my scar, the skin is becoming rather tight, I'm experiencing a good bit of pressure, my foobies are no longer symmetrical, I have a sore throat, and a metallic taste in my mouth. Since the skin is becoming tight, my range of motion is also limited, and doing my physical therapy exercises is rather painful. The radiation has been making me extremely fatigued as well. I go for treatment at 8:30 am, then go home for a two-hour nap, go to work, and then sleep through the night. I'm not complaining though because I'm catching up on all the sleep I missed out on for the past five months. Despite all of the side effects, I'm focusing on the positive...in five more days, I will not be a hairy, smelly cancer patient anymore. Hello Bic shaver and deodorant!!

I'm not sure what happens when the radiation is finished, but I will be making an appointment to see my plastic surgeon for him to check the effects of the radiation on the skin and implant.

Wednesday, October 3, 2007
Radiation: Mission Complete!

Tuesday, October 2nd was my thirtieth and final radiation treatment. It was a bitter-sweet feeling. I so anxiously wanted it to be over, but there is a part of me that is a little nervous about not having someone watching over me. I have been under the watchful eye of my doctors for the past six months, so I kind of having this feeling of "now what?"

I think a lot of my anxiety comes from the fact that in October 2006 when I went for my yearly exam, there wasn't a lump, and four months later, there it was at 1cm and less than two months after that, it grew to 2cm. And with knowing that I'm at high risk for recurrence, it only increases my anxiety. I go back for my one-month check up on November 5th. I also see the medical oncologist that day. Then I will rotate between my five doctors every three to four months for the next several years. I have to continue with my skin care for the next month but am now using Silvadene because of the burning to my scar. They said the side effects could last for another two to four weeks, but I do have nicely shaved and sweet-smelling armpits.

Wednesday, October 3, 2007
A Young Face of Breast Cancer

I went down to the North Shore today to see the fountain at Point State Park turn pink for Breast Cancer Awareness month. It was an emotional experience because I'm now part of the group no one ever signs up to be a part of and because it was yet another reminder for me that I'm "too young" for this disease. Everywhere I go, I'm the youngest breast cancer patient/survivor by at least fifteen years. It breaks my heart to be repeatedly reminded of that fact. I wanted to scream when the speaker talked about the funding of mammograms starting at the age of 40. I wanted to say, "Hello, look at me, I'm 32, still eight years away from 40, but I have it!" I take issue with the lack of consideration and acknowledgment given to those of us who are in this minority population (under the age of 40), particularly when it comes to screening methods and legislation. In my opinion, if eleven thousand women under the age of 40 are diagnosed with breast cancer just this year, we need to reconsider the idea that only women over the age of 40 should receive mammograms. Why put an age limit on something that can detect cancer early on if that is what is continuously being preached? "Early detection saves lives," yet most breast cancer in young women is found beyond what would be considered "early stage." And then there is the issue of underinsured women who are under the age of 40– they totally get screwed. Okay, I'm getting off-topic here, not to mention fired up, but hopefully, it will get you thinking about these issues. Anyway....

When the ceremony ended, I went down toward the river to take a few pictures of the fountain to include in my "breast cancer journey" scrapbook. As I was coming up the stairs, a lady approached me and asked if I was a survivor (I was wearing my pink survivor t-shirt from the Susan G. Komen Race for the Cure). I told her that I am working on six months of survival. She asked me if I would be interested in doing some modeling, to which I responded, "Absolutely." I don't know all the details as of yet, but I know it will be for something in March (my cancerversary). I couldn't help but smile the whole way home. This isn't something that I want to be modeling for, but I have been praying every day that I know what I'm supposed to do with this mess. So, if being the face of a young breast cancer patient/survivor is what it is, then so be it. And, with doing the photoshoot for a calendar last month, I have to wonder if maybe this IS what I'm meant to do with this.

Tuesday, October 9, 2007
It Never Seems to End

For the past few weeks, I have been experiencing a constant aching in my back. It's not a muscle pain but a deeper bone pain. It is mostly my middle to lower back. I have been chalking it up as another side effect from the radiation, but I figured that maybe I should call Dr. Beriwal, radiation oncologist, to find out if this is related to the radiation. What a novel idea! I know. I'm brilliant. Anyway, when I called Diane, the nurse, explained that it is not a side effect of the radiation. Okay, I was wrong. Dr. Beriwal was standing right there when she had me on the phone, so she told him about my back pain, and he has recommended that I go in for a bone scan to be on the safe side. I'm scheduled for that next Tuesday, October 16th. The nurse asked me if I was taking any medication, and I explained that I would have to be in some pretty excruciating pain to take anything. The pain fluctuates in intensity, but it is always there. I'm not willing to put anything down my throat for the sake of "putting a band-aid" on the problem.

As we ended the conversation, Diane told me, "Don't worry, honey." Ya know, it's tough not to, given my current situation. Hereditary cancer and high risk for recurrence...oh, and did I already mention cancer? My gynecologist told me not to worry, too and well, look how that ended up. I am worried because I know that cancer is not sequential, as it was once thought to be. It used to be believed that cancer would start in one location, move to the lymph nodes, and then move to other parts of the body and into the bones. The truth is that cancer can also altogether bypass the lymph nodes and attack another part of your body by traveling through the bloodstream. And one has to wonder about such things when you know that cancer has been active in your body for eight to ten years to find a 1cm tumor. Again, maybe it is a curse that I know all of what I do about cancer because it creates a little more anxiety for me, but then again, if I didn't know what I know, I probably wouldn't be as aggressive in my treatment.

You know, even after six months of all this crap, I stood in my kitchen yesterday thinking to myself "Do I really have cancer? Is this really happening to me? Have I not awakened from this nightmare yet?"

It is amazing how it doesn't get easier to deal with. The pain of it today is the same as it was six months ago. I still cry, I still don't sleep through the night, and I still want to go back to my simple pre-cancer life.

Wednesday, October 17, 2007
Bone Scan

I went for my bone scan yesterday. My friend Jenna came along with me for support. I was injected with radioactive dye at about 12:30 pm and then had to be back at 3:45 pm for the scan. We went for lunch/dinner at the Cheesecake Factory. It was so yummy, and the waiter bought me a piece of cheesecake! I called the doctor today, and everything looks clear with the bone scan, but they are still concerned with the back pain that I'm having, as it is constant and fluctuates in intensity. I spoke with the doctor who assured me that it was not due to the radiation. He recommended I go in for an MRI, so I have that scheduled for this Saturday at 1pm.

I'm going to buy a t-shirt that I found online last night that says, "Please excuse the mess, I'm under construction. "Oh, how true that is– not only physically, but emotionally and mentally, as well.

Monday, October 22, 2007
I am My Own Worst Enemy

I often think back to a few days after my diagnosis when I was standing in my office with two of the secretaries that work in my department, crying and asking, "Who is going to love me now?" Those words still weigh heavily on my mind.

I find myself being very backward, intimidated, and uncomfortable in social situations where I used to be outgoing and confident. I never had a problem with approaching a man that I wanted to talk to, but I now find myself shying away from most of them, especially if there is a real possibility that something could develop. I have such overwhelming anxiety over the idea of meeting a man and eventually having to share my story with him. I'm not ashamed by any means that I'm fighting this battle. However, I can't even begin to wrap my mind around how heavy of a burden it might be on someone my age when I tell him that I have genetic breast cancer, that I'm at risk for recurrence, that I need to have my ovaries removed by the time I'm 35 years old, that I will be in pre-mature menopause, and that I'm not willing to have children despite very much wanting to have them. It is a heavy burden for me. Why would anyone else willingly want to carry such a burden? When I look at myself, all I see is how broken I am on the outside and inside. I have my doubts that I will ever love myself enough to let someone else love me, which is what scares me the most. If I can't get past what I see on the outside to what is truly on the inside, how I can expect that of another? If my own mortality has scared me, I can only imagine how it scares others. If I have significant issues with having been robbed of part of my femininity (and eventually being robbed of it all), how can I expect someone else to accept it? I have heard a thousand times how if someone loves me, he will accept me for who I am, but that is so much easier to say and believe when you are sitting on the outside of my inside.

The lyrics from the song Broken by Wideawake are a perfect expression of how I feel...

> What if I stumble, what if I fall? What if I'm the champion of the crawl and what if I lie just to cover the truth? And what if I waste all the days of my youth? And what if I cast all my dreams in the sea? What if my greatest fear is me? Where can I run to escape from this hell? Would you be there, would you be there?

> Cardiac arrest, heart pounding out of my chest, don't want to become like a crash test dummy. If I let you down, will you still want me around? If I'm broken, will you still love me?

80

What if I staple or color my skin, and what if I enjoy all of my sin? And what if I run just to hide from the noise? What if I like girls, what if boys? And what if I listen to all that they say. I promise forever and then walk away. Where can I run to escape from myself? Would you be there, would you be there?

You're so unpredictable. Your love, so unconditional, yeah but tell me, will I be alright if I don't like myself?

What if I stumble, what if I fall? What if I'm the champion of the crawl? All that I can hope for, all I can be, all I can offer you is me.

Would you still love me, if I'm broken?

What if I'm broken? Will you still love me then?

That's all I need to know, is will you still love me?

Will you still love me, if I'm broken?

Tuesday, November 6, 2007
My Body, My Life, MY DECISIONS!

Yesterday I went for my one-month follow-up with my Dr. Beriwal, my radiation oncologist, and my post-radiation appointment with my medical oncologist, Dr. Lembersky.

Dr. Beriwal was pleased that the skin has returned to its normal color but recognized that there is some tightening of the implant (to say the least, in my opinion). I will see him again in a year. I immediately left his office and went to see my medical oncologist, Dr. Lembersky.

For some reason, I had a gut feeling that I was going to leave upset after this appointment. At first, all seemed to go well, but then Dr. Lembersky questioned why I went for a bone scan and an MRI due to the back pain. He said, "You need to work through your anxieties that every little ache and pain is cancer. Estrogen positive cancer doesn't come back in two months, six months, two years, or four years." If it had been a "minor" ache or pain, I wouldn't have put myself through that, but it has been so intense at times that I was brought to my knees. But apparently, he is the cancer God!?

As if that didn't have me upset enough, he had to bring up what I dread talking about the most– MY ovaries. Why does everyone want to know if I have decided when to have my ovaries removed? I'm not ready to make that decision right now. It is a big decision to make, and honestly, I think I have been through enough physical, emotional, and mental trauma in the last six months. I'm barely through and have not even begun to digest the breast cancer issue, yet I'm being pushed into having to make another decision that I should not have to make at my age or ever for that matter. He said, "If I were you, I would take the Tamoxifen for the next five years, get married and have a baby." I told him that I'm not sure I want to have a baby. I mean, I do, but I have a hard time putting an innocent life at risk for this deadly disease. His response to that was, "Well, my father had heart disease, and he still had me." I wasn't seeing how cancer and heart disease could even be compared. I can't imagine why anyone would knowingly put an innocent life at risk, especially when cancer is involved. If I were to have a child, statistically he/she could get cancer at a much younger age than me, possibly ten years younger. Really, how could I do that? It's not like this is an easy decision for me or that it makes me very marketable in the dating scene, but I whole-heartedly do not believe I can be that selfish.

Does he think that it was easy to look at my mom and dad when I told them of my decision? Does he think it is easy for me to imagine the day when I have to tell someone about my decision and hope that he doesn't walk out of my life? It's not easy at all! It tears my heart to pieces every time I think about it.

Aside from the whole genetic factor, why in the world would I get pregnant and have estrogen hijack my body when I spent the previous five years taking an anti-estrogen pill? That makes no damn sense to me at all. I think he sensed my agitation and honestly, I should have said something, but I didn't because I get so emotional over it and I don't want him or anyone else to see how painful this is for me. I go back to see him in six months. Oh, joy!

I believe there is a saying that goes something like "All that is well ends well." I would have to think that the opposite of that would be true...All that is not well does not end well. My day started off bad with the doctor's appointment and ended badly when a 7-year old student punched the left foobie.

This day would be one that I'd like to give back. Why can't we have "do-overs"? I was so emotionally exhausted that I passed out at about 9:00 pm, and that NEVER happens.

Sunday, November 18, 2007
Thanksgiving

As the Thanksgiving holiday quickly approaches, I have been pondering what it is that I'm thankful for this year. I've never been big on the Thanksgiving tradition, but this year is obviously very different for me. I often spend time reflecting on the past six months and realize there is so much to be thankful for through this life-altering journey. This has been the most challenging and trying time in my life without a shadow of a doubt, but I'm grateful that I'm still here to see my way through this journey. I have been given a second chance at life, something some others have not been provided for reasons that I will never understand. I'm thankful for every single breath I can breathe, every morning that I wake up to see a new day and every moment that I'm able to live. I'm thankful that, as of right now, I have cheated death. I'm grateful that I'm still here to feel joy, love, sorrow, and pain, and to be able to appreciate all of those feelings. I'm thankful that I have been given the opportunity to right the wrongs in my life.

I am not perfect by any means, and I have made huge mistakes- some I'm not very proud of- but I have the chance to learn from those mistakes and not repeat them. I'm thankful that I can still strive to achieve my goals of making a difference, changing a life, and touching a heart so that when I am gone from this world, that will be part of the legacy I leave behind. I'm thankful I'm able to see the world (and my life) through an entirely new perspective. Life is a precious gift that should not be wasted or taken for granted. I'm thankful I have learned who and what is truly important in this life and that the most important things in life are not "things" at all. I'm thankful I have my three precious, little nieces that look up to me and love me with all of their hearts. I'm grateful I can play a part in shaping who they become as teenagers and young adults. I'm thankful I have parents who love me to no end and are proud of all that I have done. I'm grateful I have a support system of family and friends who have stood by my side throughout this entire journey and have shown me how much I am truly loved. I'm thankful for all of those who have reached out to touch my hand but touched my heart instead. I'm grateful for all of the ways that cancer has changed the core of who I am. Though I do not like what I see on the outside, the person on the inside of this is a much more loving, kind, and compassionate person than ever before. I'm thankful for all of the ways I have turned this life-shattering experience into something positive- the calendar, modeling for Tickle Me Pink in March, telling my story, being a part of the Teens for the Cure at my school, supporting women with breast cancer, and volunteering my time.

As you sit around the dinner table with your family and friends and are asked what you are thankful for on Thanksgiving, I hope you realize there is so much to be grateful for in all of our lives, no matter how challenging

84

things may be or how unfair and unjust life can be at times. We all have the gift of life and love, and the most precious gifts are the ones that do not come with a price tag.

I got this quote from my sweet Kyle, who is very dear to my heart and has seen his fair share of unjust in this world, but still finds a way to smile and enjoy life.

"When my time is up, and I stand before my maker, I'd like to be able to say, "God, I don't have one ounce of talent, love, compassion or energy left. I used every gift you gave me." -Unknown

Tuesday, November 27, 2007
Emerald Dream Ball Princess

I had entered the Emerald Dream contest at the beginning of November for which I had to write a thousand-word essay about my breast cancer experience. It was a national search for twelve women with a compelling breast cancer story, and the grand prize is an all-expenses-paid trip to Las Vegas from December 26 through January 2, 2008, for a week of pampering- makeup, hair, and wardrobe makeovers, spa treatments, and much, much more. The twelve women chosen will receive a tailor-made evening gown and will be featured in a theatrical production on New Year's Eve called the Emerald Dream Ball, which will be attended by celebrities, and there will be male models, as well. Woo Hood! As if all of that isn't enough, the whole thing is being filmed by Lifetime Movie Network and will be aired as, "Top This Party." I received some exciting news on November 21st at 7 pm as I was packing for my mini-vacation to Arizona. I picked up the phone, thinking it was going to be my dad wondering why I wasn't home yet, but it was not. The woman asked if I was Melissa Ward and then identified herself as Jen from Emerald Dream. I gasped the biggest gasp ever and then she told me I won. I began jumping up and down, squealing, "I WON, I WON, I WON." I was in complete hysterics for some time after that and couldn't wait to tell everyone. I'm headed to Las Vegas for my Christmas break to live like a princess for a week!

Wednesday, December 12, 2007
Leaving the Door Open

For those who have kept up to date on my cancer journey, they know how devastating it has been for me to accept the decision I made to give up having children. That decision alone was probably one of the single most heart-wrenching for me. Well, being one that never stops thinking, I may have come up with a way to leave that door open. After much careful thought and consideration, I have decided to meet with a fertility specialist to discuss what options are actually available to me if I should choose to have children. My idea may vary from what is actually scientifically possible, but I don't think I'm too far off on this one. I'm going to harvest some of my eggs so that they are readily available, if and when the time would come that those eggs would need to be used.

There is a process already in practice that the genetic makeup of a particular egg can be examined and since we know that my mutation is at chromosome 13, it could easily be determined if that egg carries that same mutation. If the genetic variation is present, the egg is tossed. An egg that does not have the genetic mutation can be artificially inseminated, and one would then become impregnated through in-vitro fertilization. Since my cancer is estrogen positive, the last thing I want to do is to let estrogen hijack my body by getting pregnant. Though I don't think there would be any greater joy in this world than carrying my own child, I can't take the risk of not making it through the pregnancy to mother a child. SO, I would look at finding someone to be a surrogate for me. This at least gives me some hope that seeing a little Melissa sometime in the future is still possible. What a gift that child would be, not only for me, but for so many in my life. Of course, this is all in my head, but I will know more once I'm able to meet with the fertility specialist. So...I'm currently accepting applications for a surrogate since I would prefer it be someone that I know. Though I'm nowhere near this stage of my life, I'm going to be proactive in this so that I can't look back and say, if only I had...

Also, I switched to a different medical oncologist. I will now be working with a female. I'm hoping that she will be a little more sensitive to the issues I'm facing and won't say "Hello, Beautiful" every time she sees me.

14 more days until Vegas!! Yeah, Baby!

Wednesday, January 2, 2008
Happy New Year!

Happy 2008! I hope this year is full of beautiful things. I'm looking forward to a new beginning and starting my journey beyond my breast cancer experience. I had an exciting and extravagant start to 2008, so I'm hoping that is how the rest of my year will go. Vegas was quite the experience, and I had fun despite all of the chaos, frustration, disorganization, and stress. I enjoyed being in the spotlight and put my face in front of the cameras every chance I could.

However, the Emerald Dream Ball was not the highlight of my trip. The best part of my trip was seeing someone after ten years who has held a very special place in my heart for a very long time. I met Justin eleven years ago at Cedar Point, where we both were working for the summer. He had recently graduated from high school, and I was entering my senior year of college the following fall. We had spent almost every single day together after we met. There were many late nights at the local grocery store, restaurants, and bars. No matter what we did, where we went, or whom we were with, Justin and I always had a great time. He became my best friend, and I became his. It was apparent to everyone that as we grew closer together, our hearts did as well, and eventually, we ended up falling in love with each other. Though I think he knew how I felt, and I knew how he felt, we never told the other about our feelings until it was too late. I remember going to his dorm the night before he left to say goodbye and give him a present. I gave him a framed picture of me from my 21st birthday, the song Nobody Knows by The Tony Rich Project, and a letter telling him how much I loved him. I cried for hours on end after I knew he was gone. We maintained minimal contact throughout the next year, and when I returned to Cedar Point the following year, I had a boyfriend. Justin and I grew apart that summer; everything had changed. I don't even remember saying goodbye to him. We continued to drift apart, and there were years that we didn't even talk. I had tracked him down through his father twice and then found him on MySpace.

When I found out that I would be going to Las Vegas, where he lives now, I was ecstatic over the idea of being able to see him after all these years. The first night I was there, I did exactly that. We only had 10 minutes together that night because he was working. We were able to manage some time together two other days while I was there and despite having not seen each other for so long, it was like we had never missed a beat. Everything was the same as it had always been between us. We had a blast in downtown Vegas. We rode the Big Shot at the top of the Stratosphere. The following day, we met up again for a late lunch/early dinner. That evening, he gave me a script for a movie that he had written about our summer together.

Before he got to my hotel, I read the script and cried that we both let go of one another. While at the restaurant, I kept thinking to myself how hard it was going to be for me to let go of him again. He dropped us off at the hotel and got out of the car to give me a hug and say goodbye. We stood there for what seemed like an eternity hugging one another. I didn't want to let go of him. I don't think he realized that I was crying until he let go a bit and looked at me. He hugged me again, and I buried my head into his chest and cried harder. I made him walk away from me because I couldn't do it again. It took everything in me to walk into the hotel as he drove away. I guess there was a part of me that was hoping that things would have changed after all of these years, that it would be awkward to be around each other because things were different. That wasn't the case, and that made it all the harder to walk away from him again. Though we promised that it would not be 10 years before we saw each other again, I have cried numerous tears at the thought that it may have been the last time I ever see him.

Sunday, January 6, 2008
Just for a Minute

The last two days have been rather difficult and trying for me. I spent many hours lying in bed this weekend with the blankets over my head pondering one of my life's greatest mysteries...my cancer. I still have not yet begun to understand how this is/could be the reality of my life. I lie there in bed saying to myself "I'm 32 and I have cancer! I'm 32, and I have cancer?" Amazing how it never gets any easier to say those words; the pain still stings the same as it did before. As I lie there, I wished that for one minute, the world around me would stop, or maybe slow down a bit. I don't understand how this all happened so fast– it will soon be a year since I received the news that devastated me and changed my life forever. I feel like I have lost so much time—precious time—because of all of this; time that I will never get back.

I feel like, there were so many things I should have been doing instead of spending my time worrying about the next devastating blow, wondering if I would see tomorrow, recovering from one surgery after another, and putting my body and mind through pure hell. I think I was so busy going through the motions that I never gave myself a chance to understand what was happening to me. Honestly, I still don't think that the full impact of what I have been through has hit me. What a joyful day that will be when it finally does.

Then I started thinking about how in less than a year, my body and my perceptions of it changed significantly. It has been an ongoing struggle for me to come to terms with giving up a part of what defines me as a woman, but now I'm also dealing with how the radiation has impacted the foobies. The right side has become hard and so tight that I have a hard time stretching my arm over my head. I can't keep my bra centered and am constantly fidgeting with and readjusting it. I was hoping the tissue wouldn't shrink and the implant wouldn't harden. I hoped that for once, I would be the minority in a positive way. I'm frustrated that I will have to undergo surgery to remove tissue from my back to put under the foobie as the right side is about an inch higher than the left at this point. To add more insult to injury, the full effects of radiation may not be evident for six months to a year after the last treatment. So, I am left wondering when I will be able to have the surgery.

How many times can I be ripped apart and sewn back together? I feel like someone's old teddy bear that had its limbs taken off and then hand-stitched back on. Then I remembered that in two and a half years, I will have to undergo another surgery- more ripping apart and sewing me back together. I will be a walking Frankenstein. I already loathe looking in the mirror, and there are only more scars that I will have to carry soon, not only on the outside but also on the inside. If I could heal the wounds on the inside, maybe, just maybe, I could handle those on the outside. I wish that for a minute I could step away from myself to make the pain go away, to wipe the tears from my eyes, to have the heartache cease, and to not face this cruel beast on my own day in and day out. Then as I remember that the world and life continue to go on while I'm trying to hide from it. I drag myself out of bed and think about the song What I Cannot Change by Leann Rimes.

I will learn to let go of what I cannot change, I will learn to forgive what I cannot change, I will learn to love what I cannot change. I will change whatever I can.

Saturday, January 12, 2008
Treatment Update

I met with my new medical oncologist, Dr. Shannon Puhalla, on Monday, January 7th for a consultation. We reviewed my cancer journey from the beginning to the present. I like her, and she seemed very interested in knowing my whole history. She didn't minimize the genetic mutation or question my decision regarding children. Nor did she ask why I have not yet decided to have my ovaries removed. She offered medication to control the hot flashes from the Tamoxifen, but I expressed my disinterest in taking an anti-depressant for that. I'm not one to medicate myself, so I will suck it up as I have been. I had some blood drawn for the clinical trial while I was there. Overall, it was a very uneventful appointment. I scheduled an appointment with Dr. Gimbel, my plastic surgeon, on Wednesday, January 9th, as I had a little bit of a "scare" this week. On Monday evening, I found a "lump" along the top edge of the right foobie. It feels very much like the tumor did, so I wasn't willing to brush it off. I called the plastic surgeon on Tuesday to schedule an appointment, and luckily, they were able to get me in the next day to be seen. Of course, like last time, I didn't tell a whole lot of people because I didn't want to scare anyone or have anyone say that I was over-reacting. It most certainly had me on edge and took me right back to February 20, 2007 when I found my tumor. It was hard not to think about the worst-case scenario when I had heard a thousand times before that it was going to be okay and that it probably wasn't cancer...then the bomb was dropped on me that it was.

To my relief, the plastic surgeon told me that he thinks it is a wrinkle in the implant. I knew that it was possible with all of the changes that are taking place on that side, however; I'm still going to monitor it for any signs of growth. He did say that it seemed as though the right side was being affected by the radiation, and I laughed at him and said, "It seems?" He asked me if it is obvious when I'm wearing a bra, and I explained the whole problem with it always shifting to the left side. Then I told him about my trying on a corset the day before. Wow was that funny. Not really, but what else could I do but laugh? The difference between the two implants was SO noticeable that I stood in the dressing room laughing at myself for about five minutes and saying, "This is so fucked up. Seriously, this is so fucked up."

He suggested that my next surgery be completed in April/May to fix the skin under the implant, though there are no guarantees that the skin won't shrink again, and I may have to undergo yet another surgery to fix it again. Boo! The good news is that he gave me clearance to go skydiving before my next surgery, so I'm planning another jump in early to mid-April!

92

Tuesday, January 22, 2008
Too Funny Not to Share

I had been planning on getting a tattoo of the FORCE (Facing Our Risk of Cancer Empowered) heart, which is half of a pink ribbon and half of a teal ribbon, since I found out the cancer is genetic. It represents hereditary breast and ovarian cancer. Yesterday was the day! My friend Annette and I went down to the tattoo shop, and I did it. The whole experience of getting the tattoo was uneventful, but I think I figured out why a lot of my friends seem to enjoy those vibrating toys. Anyway, the best part of the tattoo experience was the lady who noticed the little handcuff pin on my jacket and insisted on showing me something that I "would just love." She showed me a set of handcuffs that are meant for pierced nipples. It was rather interesting...a handcuff for each nip and then a chain connecting them. I made a statement about how nice they were while I thought to myself, "Self, how would that work for me? It would sure be interesting." She then commented that when I decide to get my nipples pierced, I could get that. Annette and I looked at one another and laughed. I said, "Yeah, I'm going to get MY nipples pierced." As the tattoo artist continued to prepare for my tattoo, Annette and I continued to talk to this lady. Throughout our conversation, she made reference to my getting my nipples pierced two other times. Finally, on the third time that she had made a comment and as she was answering the phone, I blurted out, "I don't have any nipples!" The look on her face was priceless. I think I was in a little bit of shock that I actually said it too. Had she left well enough alone, I wouldn't have felt the need to clear the air about it, but she wouldn't let it go. We continued to laugh about it after that. I kind of felt bad for her because I'm sure she doesn't see very many 32 year-olds coming through there that don't have nipples. She did offer to surface pierce the foobies, and as "appealing" as that seems, I think I will pass on that. I already look like a freak...let's not kick it up a notch. I'm glad I was able to find the humor in the whole thing because there most certainly was a time (and there are still days) I would have responded differently.

Tuesday, February 5, 2008
Same Old Yesterday

It's 5:00 am when the alarm clock goes off. I lie there in a daze listening and internally singing along to Everybody by Keith Urban, which is one of my "cancer comfort" songs. The lyrics of the song strike a chord deep within me, shaking the core of my very being.

> So here you are now, nowhere to turn. It's just the same old yesterday. You made a promise to yourself that you were never gonna be this way. And the only thing that you've ever known is to run, so you keep on driving faster into the sun. But everybody needs somebody sometimes. Yeah, everybody needs somebody sometimes. Don't have to find your own way out. You got a voice, let it be heard. Just when it feels you're on a dead-end road, there's always somewhere left to turn. So don't give up to now, you're so close to a brand new day. Yes, you are. And if you just can't bear to be alone, I'll stay cuz everybody needs somebody sometimes. Everybody needs somebody sometimes. Well, baby, I've been too caught up to see what you've been going through. All I can say is I'm here now. And everybody needs somebody sometimes.

As I absorb every word of the song, I start to cry quietly. The tears begin to fall harder and faster as I think about having nowhere to turn, and every day since March 15, 2007 has been the same old yesterday. Nothing seems to have changed except that I've lost myself through all of this. I'm always trying to run away from all of this– the anger, the hurt, the pain, the tears, the hopelessness– with nowhere to go.

I think of how tired I am of battling this head-on every day by myself. I wish that for one day, I could wake up to hear this song in the arms of somebody and feel a level of comfort that would get me through the day. Somebody that could make the world seem okay...slow it down a little bit and help me to see the world and life differently because it doesn't look so great through my own eyes. Then I feel myself getting pissed off that I could be so selfish to want to bring someone into my living hell. Any thought I had about needing someone has been completely wiped away. I think to myself that I will never bring anyone into this, not because I don't need someone, but because that someone does not need this.

The song ends, and I hit the snooze button, hoping that another nine minutes will somehow change something, anything. The alarm goes off again. I get up to go do one of my two workouts for the day because it's something, possibly the only thing, that I feel I have any control over. I finish and go shower to start my day. I undress out of sight from the mirror so that I don't have to look at what I hate so much. I get out of the shower and immediately robe myself without looking. I sit down in front of my

94

mirror to start my daily routine. I think about how much I miss my "old" body and look up at the pictures I had taken the day before my mastectomy as I push back the tears that so desperately want to fall. Then I look at what I have "become"– the harsh reality of what this disease has done to me. The anger starts to build as I look at not only the five scars I carry, but also the impact of the radiation. I cover myself back up and finish my routine.

I begin to shuffle through my clothes in my closet to find something to wear that will mask the very obvious asymmetrical foobies. I change two or three times until I find something that might work, but then I think if I remember to keep my hair draping over them, no one will be able to tell, or so I think. I leave the apartment, coaching myself the whole way to work that I can get through today. "Just let me get through today, and I will worry about tomorrow when it comes."

It takes every last bit of my energy to get through the day without breaking down, often to the point of exhaustion. Every time someone asks me how I'm doing; I push back the urge to say what I'm really feeling. I simply give them a fake smile and say I'm fine. This is how my entire day goes.

Finally, it's time to go home, but I don't want to go because there is nothing there. I've jam-packed my weeknights with different activities but mostly working out, so I go to the gym and get in my second workout for the day. Afterward, I go home, and the best I can hope for is that someone will call or text me, or maybe someone sent me some mail. Most days, it's none of the above. I occupy myself by doing more work at home until I have nothing left in me and then make my way to bed. I'm able to sleep for only a little bit at a time. Each time I wake up, my mind races a thousand miles a minute. The next thing I know...it's 5 am, and the alarm clock goes off. I lie there again, listening and internally singing along to Everybody by Keith Urban.

Thursday, February 14, 2008
Love and All that Crazy Stuff

Today is a day that I typically dread and have for a very long time. I've had so many horrible experiences with Valentine's Day throughout my adult life that it's just another day for me. "A big marketing scheme," is how I've always viewed it. One day this week, Justin sends me a text message asking where I work on Thursday and being the clueless person that I am, I thought to myself, "Why would he be asking this? He must have accidentally texted the wrong person." I reply, telling him that I work in the same place every day, my office at school, and why in the world is he asking. As I'm texting him, I'm talking on the phone with my mom who reminds me that it's Valentine's Day on Thursday. Oh!

We exchanged a few other text messages before he asked for my school address, so I told him, "You're not getting it unless you are what is being delivered." Very cute, I know. I'm witty like that! He didn't particularly like that response, so I caved and gave him the address.

As I was sitting in my office at work, one of the guys comes in with a big red box. He tells me it had been sitting downstairs for two weeks before they finally tracked it down to me. That totally threw me off, the math wasn't adding up in my head. I'm sitting here thinking, "So, if this isn't from Justin, then who is it from, and why would I want them after they have been sitting somewhere for two weeks?" Then the guy laughs and tells me that he got them today. As I'm opening them up, the two secretaries who were with me the day I got my diagnosis and have seen me shed tears as I talk about how nobody will ever love me came in to see what was going on. My body temperature rose to what felt like 200 degrees. I don't know if I was blushing or having a hot flash. I suspect I was blushing. Sure enough, Justin sent me a beautiful bouquet of red, pink, yellow, and purple roses and some Godiva chocolate. This girl is glowing on the inside and the outside. The smile on my face is genuine for once and is bigger than it has been in a very long time.

Thursday, February 14, 2008
Tickle Me Pink

My day keeps getting better! As if I wasn't already beaming with joy, I received a phone call from Susan G. Komen about the Tickle Me Pink luncheon on March 9th. I will be one of the models for the event! So now I have two reasons to be smiling from ear-to-ear, and I am indeed!

Wednesday, February 20, 2008
Discovery Day

So here it is...February 20th, the day that I discovered my tumor. I remember it so vividly that it's like it happened yesterday.

For the past few weeks, I've had a tough time thinking about dealing with this day. It carries so many different emotions for me that I feel like I'm on a rollercoaster with many dips, turns, and loops. My anxiety has increased tenfold, and my emotions are on overdrive. There is this constant swirling of emotions in my head and deep within my soul because I'm both saddened and happy over what this day means to me. This day marks two significant events. The first is my discovery day, also known as the start of my living hell. It is the day that everything in my life as I knew it started to change, and the downward spiral began

It is also the birthday of one of my very best friends and the person I call my co-survivor, Ken. I can't even begin to explain to you how instrumental this person has been in my journey through the cancer world. He is one of the very few people that will talk to me openly and honestly about my cancer. He has walked side-by-side with me throughout this journey, has picked me up when I have fallen, and has pushed me forward when I have felt like I couldn't do it anymore. Simply stated, he is nothing short of amazing.

The weekend before my third surgery (July 16th), I wrote a poem for him. I have only shared it with my other best friend. In honor of his birthday, I want to share it so you can understand how truly amazing and wonderful my co-survivor is.

CO-SURVIVOR

From the day that I was diagnosed with breast cancer, you never pretended to have or be able to find the answers.

When you have a hard time finding the right words to say, "ROCK ON, WARD" is all I need to make my day.

You wear your pin, necklace, and pink bracelet each day, to show the world that you support me all the way.

You always look beyond that beautiful and often fake smile, in hopes that you will understand and feel my pain once in a while.

You are my strength when I do not have enough to get through the day, and you are always here to pick me up when I fall along the way.

With me, you laugh and with me, you cry and I know you will continue to be my "rock" when I question why.

You have helped me to see that through the rain I must go if at the end of this journey I want to find my rainbow.

For the time we have known each other, you have been a very dear friend. I do not know that I would get through this without you here to walk with me to the end.

Close to my heart is where you shall remain forever because you have been more than just a friend-

You are my CO-SURVIVOR.

With all true meanings of the words, Your Friend,
Melissa

Sunday, February 24, 2008
Our Supermodel Society

From the time we are little people, we are faced with images of what defines a woman or a man, especially attractive women and men. I remember being a teenager and wanting to look like Cindy Crawford. I was envious because she had it all– long legs, a rockin' body, and a gorgeous face. I never imagined that at the age of 32, I would be thinking those same thoughts all over again. But....

It's Friday evening, and I have finally decided to leave work at about 6:15 pm to go be the lame person I have become through all of this cancer crap. As I'm making the turn onto the street before my apartment, I hear an advertisement on the radio that I have heard a thousand times before, but for whatever reason, it hit me hard on this particular day. It goes something like "Attention women 18 years or older who have ever considered breast enhancement surgery. Get the big, full, incredibly sexy breasts you have always wanted. Get the attention-getting body and breasts you deserve." I could have easily turned the station and ignored this stupid advertisement, but no, I decide to torture myself. The only thing I keep hearing over and over throughout the minute and a half is "incredibly sexy breasts." I find myself becoming extremely irritated because it only validates my belief that society is overly obsessed with boobs, and well, mine have been ripped away from me. Not that they were much to brag about before all of this, but they were mine, and I liked them. Then I start thinking about my friend who got her breast enhancement surgery right around the time that I made the decision to have my bilateral mastectomy. She went to my appointment with me the day I met with my surgical oncologist, which was one of the worst things I could have done to myself. There she was flashing me her newly enhanced D cups in her low-cut shirt, and I was sobbing that in a few weeks I would be robbed of my own to be replaced with the foreign objects. I was angry and frustrated that she had a choice, and I didn't. I remember contemplating digging my eyes out with pencils or stabbing her new implants so that they would deflate. I still have my eyes. She still has her Ds.

After a few minutes of sitting in the car outside my apartment on the verge of tears, I go inside. As I sift through my mail, I find two of the ten or so Victoria Secret's catalogs that I get in a week. I honestly don't know why I don't toss them in the trash the moment I get them, but I look through them. Most times, I can honestly say that it isn't because I'm going to buy something but instead looking at the pictures and wishing so much that I could have back what used to be mine. Instead, I have these things inside of me that will never truly be a part of me. I guess the only way I can think to explain what it is like would be for you to imagine having your entire arm fall asleep. You know how it doesn't feel like it is a part of you, that's how the foobies feel. The difference is that you eventually get the feeling back in your arm...for me, this feeling is there 24/7, and it's not a pins and needles kind of sensation, it's no feeling. I realize that I have become somewhat obsessed with breasts, not in a sexual way; more like I had them, but now they are gone, and that makes me less desirable, less beautiful, less sexy...less of a woman. The women in the catalog have nice perfectly shaped boobs, and here mine are, a diagonal scar across both of them, missing nipples, mismatched and asymmetrical (one looks like a mini basketball and the other looks like a baseball). Ah yes, I have revisited my dreadful teenage years. While I know that most of the population does not look like Cindy Crawford, it is a much different kind of envy when you have had something taken away from you against your will. Though I have heard people tell me a million times how beautiful I am, it is still hard to feel differently than I do when images of what society tells me I should look like are constantly being shoved in my face.

Sunday, March 9, 2008
Tickled Pink Tea

Today was the Tickled Pink Tea sponsored by the Susan G. Komen Foundation. I modeled for Coldwater Creek. I walked around the event and talked to the women that were interested in purchasing the outfit. Previously, they presented a runway show, but that changed this year. Several vendors were selling pink ribbon items. I found t-shirts for my three nieces, so I went back to the room to get my purse. When I entered the room, a lady asked me if I would mind being interviewed for the Ford Pink Warrior project. I excitedly said, "Of course, I would love to." The video will be shown on the Susan G. Komen website, aired the day of the Race for the Cure, and possibly be part of the Ford commercials.

The lady asked me several questions. The first question she asked was about the day of my diagnosis and how I felt. I became very emotional and told her that I was diagnosed on March 15, 2007 and would be celebrating my one-year cancerversary this week. She asked me how I'm doing today.

I was honest and said, "Okay. I still have another surgery to get through yet and the reconstruction isn't where I would like it to be, but I will get there."

The lady then asked me what makes me a believer. My response was my faith; that I have to believe that God has a plan for me through this. It is a plan for good and not for evil. Though I may not understand what his plan is right now, I know that it is something bigger than what I could even begin to imagine.

She asked me what makes me a survivor and I told her that for the longest time, I viewed it as just that...surviving. I have since learned that it's less about surviving and more about living. Getting up and facing the world each day makes me a survivor because it would be much easier to stay in bed with the blankets over my head to shut the world out and not let anyone help me through this. But I don't. I get up and I keep living. When she asked me what makes me a fighter, I struggled to keep it together. I told her it is my three nieces that make me a fighter. I can't imagine my world without them, and I can't imagine their world without me. I want to be here to see them graduate from high school and go on to college. I have to be here to watch them grow up because I will never have any children of my own.

She asked me what Susan G. Komen meant to me. It was Susan G. Komen that I had contacted first after getting my diagnosis. I had been doing the breast cancer walks for many years before my diagnosis, but it was a different feeling being on the other side of it last year. I shared that I went to the race ten days after having my bilateral mastectomy and my friend pushed me in a wheelchair all five miles. It gave me hope and strength to see so many other women facing the same disease that has shattered my life. It was a place where I didn't feel so alone and isolated; they all knew what I was going through. By the end of the interview, almost everyone in the room was in tears.

When I finished my interview, I changed my clothes and joined the rest of the ladies for the tea. The speaker was a breast cancer survivor and very funny. I felt a little out of place because as I looked around, I noticed that I was quite a bit younger than the other women. I'm not sure whether some of them realized that I, too, am a breast cancer survivor. At the end, the speaker had some of us volunteer to talk, so I stood up in front of four hundred women that I don't know and shared that Saturday is my one-year cancerversary. I told them my family and friends would be joining me for a Pink Ribbon Princess Dinner Party in a celebration of life. I said that I've learned that friends are those who reach out to touch your hand and end up touching your heart instead. Then I did the unthinkable, I said: "And I have to tell you about my nipple experience" (this was because the speaker had brought it up at one point) and told of the lady at the tattoo shop telling me about getting my nipples pierced. Everyone thought it was hysterical.

Of everything the speaker said today, there was one thing that stuck out for me- "A friend is someone who knows the song in your heart and can sing it back to you when you have forgotten how it goes." So simple, yet so profound. I'm lucky to have so many wonderful family and friends who can sing my song to me when I can't quite sing it on my own.

Wednesday, March 12, 2008
Never Ending Cancer Story

Anniversaries of any kind are emotionally charged. Today was another emotional day for me. It was one year ago today that I had my ultra-sound guided needle biopsy. I remember everything about it and thinking back to that day brings me to tears. I remember the exact outfit I was wearing and how I felt.

As I said, it was already an emotionally charged day to start. Then I had to call my plastic surgeon while I was at work because I have been experiencing significant pain in my ribs on the right side. I stopped wearing a bra some weeks ago because the pressure was too much. He wasn't sure if it is because the tissue is shrinking on that side or not but suggested that I take some Ibuprofen. I explained that I don't do that, and he said he knows. His concern is that I'm not one to readily complain about pain, so he knows that it's pretty significant. Then we got into further discussion about the implant and my upcoming surgery. He is sure he will have to remove the muscle from my back and insert a tissue expander again on the right side. This means I will have another scar on the right side of my chest and back. He said that I could look at some pictures to see what my scar will be like, but I sobbed the one and only time I tried looking at those.

During the surgery, he will swap out the left implant to put in a different implant as we had discussed before. Then in three months, I will have to go back for another surgery to have the tissue expander removed and the right implant put back in. I will be lopsided (again) for another three months. I wasn't expecting to hear that I would have to go through a second surgery. It all hit me like a ton of bricks.

I walked out to my dear friend Naomi and said, "I hate to ask this, but I need a hug." Without even a question, she stood up to hug me and let me cry. As I told her, I just want this to be over with. I know that it will never be entirely over because I have to live with this the rest of my life, but wow, I will have had five surgeries in less than a year and a half. It is physically tiring. I'm not sure how it is that I continue to function daily with being so emotionally drained.

I feel like I'm living in my NEVER-ENDING CANCER STORY.

Saturday, March 15, 2008
One-year Cancerversary

Well, here it is- my one-year cancerversary. Oh, the emotions that come with this day! There is happiness that I'm still alive to write this, but there is still the heartache and the pain that I have actually had to go through all of this. There is anger over having my dreams shattered and being robbed of a part of me. I couldn't sleep much last night as the day I got the news kept running through my head like a song on repeat.

There is a song that is part of my Cancer Comfort CD called Maybe Tonight, Maybe Tomorrow by Wideawake. The lyrics of this song are truly an expression of how I felt that day.

> I heard the news today. It came out of nowhere. Wish I could run away, but where would I go? Is this my destiny? Something to wonder...What will become of me? God only knows.

> And they say the road to heaven; it might lead us back through hell. Maybe tonight, maybe tomorrow, we'll win this fight and bury this sorrow. We're so alive, still holding on, not ready to die, so we LIVESTRONG.

> My pride is left for dead, as my world gets shaken. The thoughts inside my head so hard to control. I'm staring down the unknown. One thing for certain, it may break my body but never break my soul.

> They say the road to heaven; it might lead us back through hell so we're holding on for more than stories to tell. Maybe tonight, maybe tomorrow, we'll win this fight and bury this sorrow. We're so alive, still holding on, not ready to die, so we LIVESTRONG.

> We livestrong. We livestrong. We livestrong.

I will leave you with this poem that was given to me by my dear friend, Kathy Hahesy.

> She Who Survived

> One day she woke up, and her world changed forever.
> She was confronted with a fight for life she never dreamed she'd face.
> Miraculously, she survived.
> The battle was not easy, but she knew she'd win.
> She did everything to find a cure...
> Expanding her horizons medically and spiritually

And sharing her new-found knowledge with every woman she knows.
She will never give up...never, never, never.
Indeed, she is the epitome of a true survivor.
Not only for herself, but for all the women in her life,
She PROUDLY wears a pink ribbon.
- Suzie Toronto

Sunday, March 16, 2008
Pink Ribbon Princess Party

Yesterday, about twenty of my family and friends got together at TGIFriday for my one-year cancerversary. My best girlfriend, Chris, came down from Erie to join us for the celebration. Chris and I have been friends for nine years and have had some crazy times together, so I knew it was going to be an exciting evening. Initially, the plan was to go to Giant Eagle to get my prescription of Tamoxifen and then head over for dinner. Then, I decided that it is more important that I have a tiara for my party than my cancer meds. We went to Party City and got two crowns for the two of us and then a pack of six tiaras for anyone else at the party that wanted one. I also got a pink boa to wear.

We arrived at TGIF after most of my party was already there- a princess always makes a grand entrance! It was overwhelming emotionally to walk in and see every one of them wearing pink. We totally stood out because most of the people were wearing green in celebration of St. Patrick's Day. It was such a great time! I gave everyone a breast cancer pin and made pink ribbon cookies. My friend, Chuck, was videotaping so that my mom can take it with her when she visits my little brother in Colorado next weekend. I was, of course, preoccupied with my nieces as I always am, and got to spend very little time conversing with anyone else. Calie had to go to the potty at one point, and I took her so her mom could eat. Everyone stared and smiled at us as we walked to the restroom. We were standing at the sink, washing her hands when one of the employees asked if we were having a princess party. I smiled and said, "Kind of. We are celebrating my one-year cancerversary." She didn't know what to say and apologized for asking. I told her that it was okay, and I'm glad she asked because I want people to know that breast cancer isn't an "old lady" disease. She asked me if Calie was my baby and I told her that she is my niece but is one of the reasons why I fight so hard every day to win this battle. She started to cry, so I walked over and gave her a hug. It was the most amazing experience I've ever had in a public restroom. When I got back from the bathroom, Chuck had ordered a mudslide with two straws. SAWEET! Since I shouldn't and don't drink, he is always kind enough to order something I like so that I can take a sip. It was so good. We were at the restaurant until about 7:00 pm or so and I'm sure they were ready for us to leave. As I waited for Chris near the main entrance while she used the ladies' room, everyone kept staring and smiling at me. It humored me.

Chris and I arrived at my apartment still wearing our tiaras and got a compliment from a guy that lives in my building. We contemplated going out to the bar or staying in. Since neither of us drink, it didn't make very much sense to go to a crowded bar with a bunch of people that had probably been drinking all day just to get a glass of water, so we decided that we would go to Blockbuster to rent some videos and hang at home.

Of course, we went to get the movies while still wearing our tiaras. Everyone was staring at us there, too. I'm not sure why it is that people act like they have never seen princesses before! Some guy stopped us and informed us that we were wearing something fuzzy on our heads and then asked why. As Chris started to unbutton her sweater to show him the Save the Ta-tas t-shirt she was wearing, the man told her not to take off her clothes. He was creepy. I shared that we were having a pink ribbon princess party in celebration of my one-year cancerversary. He and his friend thought that was awesome. He said he hoped I have a hundred and twenty more cancerversaries. I said, "Dear Lord, I don't. That would make me 152 years old." Could you imagine that? Everything would be sagging except my perky silicone implants. We rented the Nanny Diaries and A Mighty Heart. We only got through the Nanny Diaries before we were both completely exhausted and had to go to bed. The best part is that we sat on the couch watching the video with our tiaras still on!

I had questioned several times if it was a good idea for me to plan this dinner party on my one-year cancerversary. I wasn't sure if I would be able to handle it. Everything that I thought was normal in my life changed in a matter of seconds that day. March 15th is the day that my "new" life and my new normal began. My life became something so unfamiliar to me, and I lost a part of who I used to be. I was no longer that fun, carefree, party girl that everyone knew and loved. I became a cancer patient that had to fight to live. There was a part of me that wanted to stay in bed with the blankets over my head and think about how much I miss what my life used to be like but then there was the other side of me that wanted to celebrate the fact that I have made it to see another year. I often say that the score is "Boobie Cancer Fighting Princess (that would be me), one and cancer, seven." The seven is representative of all the things cancer has done to me, and the one represents the most important thing I have not lost to cancer, my life. It is because I am still here one year later that I decided to go through with my party rather than stay in bed all day with the blankets over my head. And I'm so glad that I did because I had the best time!

Monday, March 24, 2008
The Plague

Well, I've fallen victim to the cold or flu that everyone else in the free world seems to have. I had been doing so well considering that everyone in my office had been out sick for several days, but I finally got the bug last week and haven't been able to shake it. I tried Dayquil capsules without much luck. A bottle of Tylenol cold in a matter of two days has done nothing except make my head a little more foggy than usual. I've been doing the Vitamin A, C, and zinc thing with little to no success. I can't tolerate the taste of cough drops anymore, so those aren't even an option for me.

For the first time in my life, I have actually tried to take care of myself so I can get over this. I actually took the day off from work on Wednesday and did nothing more than lie in bed or on the couch most of the weekend. Oddly, I haven't been sick (until now) since I was diagnosed with the "BIG" sick. Being sick makes me a bit nervous because I know my immune system isn't at a hundred percent and I haven't been able to go to the gym, so I feel like I'm allowing cancer the opportunity to strike again.

On another note, I see my plastic surgeon, Dr. Gimbel, on Wednesday afternoon so he can check out the devastating effects from the radiation and we will be scheduling my fourth surgery. At this point, the pain in the implant and in my ribs is almost intolerable. I feel like I'm having muscle spasms again because every so often I get excruciating, sharp pains up through the implant and I'm convinced that any amount of pressure on my ribs is going to cause them to crack. Even wearing a bra causes too much pain to bear. I'm not sure how much more the implant can possibly shrink or where it will go. I have this recurring image of the implant being in my throat before I actually go in for surgery! Every day it gets a little higher and tighter. I have been trying to do some physical therapy exercises on my own because my range of motion on my right arm isn't where it should be at this point (again)...all those weeks of physical therapy for nothing!

Wednesday, March 26, 2008
One Hell of a Storm

I had my appointment with Dr. Gimbel, my plastic surgeon, today for him to examine the impact of the radiation on the implant and to plan for my upcoming surgery. He seemed taken aback by the difference between the right and left sides and the difference from the time he had seen me in January. The skin under the implant has shrunk, but the skin on the side of the implant has also shrunk, so that means the right implant is higher than the left one and narrower...significantly. I wasn't exaggerating when I said the left side looks like half of a mini basketball and the right side looks like a baseball. He suspects the tissue will continue to shrink up until the day of my surgery...oh, joy!

We talked about the two different surgery options to fix the problem. The first is less invasive and would not require having to use my latissimus muscle from my back, but it would only be a short-term fix. Dr. Gimbel said that there would be an eighty percent chance for another surgery (not counting the second one we already know I will have to undergo). The second option is to take all of my latissimus muscle on the right side of my back and pull it around to the front. Dr. Gimbel is unsure if he will be able to add that muscle around the scar area so he suspects that he will have to place it under the implant, which means that my skin there will probably be discolored, and I will have another scar.

The scar on my back from where he will take the latissimus muscle will be about six inches. This surgery is more of a long-term fix, but of course, it is not guaranteed that I won't have problems in the future. He will take the implant out on the right side and re-insert a tissue expander. I will have to get "pumped up" again, and I will still be asymmetrical until I undergo surgery in August. I opted for the second procedure because I'm not into anything short-term at this point; I want a more permanent solution. I want the poking, prodding, stabbing, ripping apart, and sewing back together to be done. I was pretty good with keeping my emotions in check during this visit considering I have only made it through one appointment without crying. I became teary-eyed at one point during our conversation, but no tears ever fell from my eyes. I was so proud of myself for having made it through the second appointment without bursting into tears...but that was quickly shattered.

When we finished with my appointment, I went to schedule the surgery with the nurse. I will be going in on May 6th (three days after my surgery last year and five days before the Susan G. Komen Race for the Cure, which means I will be in a wheelchair AGAIN!!!!! UGH!) at UPMC Shadyside. I assumed that the procedure was going to be done on an outpatient basis and never even thought to ask Dr. Gimbel. I asked the nurse about follow-up appointments so that I can make plans with my family to get me there. What she said next totally floored me and the tears flowed from my eyes and down my cheeks. She said that I would be spending at least two nights in the hospital and that I would have JP drains again. I couldn't even say anything because I was dumbfounded. She asked me if there was anything that she could do for me and I simply smiled at her and said, "No, unless you can take this all away. But thank you." She gave me the paperwork that I need to have completed before my surgery, and I left, still in tears.

As I walked to my car, I kept thinking how wrong it is that I have to go through this and I have to do it alone, at that. I cried the whole way from the doctor's office to work. I didn't want to go back to work...I was having one of those "pull the blankets over my head" moments, but I had so much that I needed to get done, I had to go back. As much as I tried to pull myself together before I got through the doors, I couldn't. I spent some time talking with three of the ladies that work in the office before I was able to pull myself back together enough to do any work.

When all of this started, there was a breast cancer survivor that said, "Honey, give it a year, and it will all be over with." I held onto that, thinking that it would be true for me. As I check the date on my watch, it is now a year and 11 days since my diagnosis, and it isn't over with. I don't know when/if it will be "over." I think that it may get easier as time passes but I'm not entirely convinced that this will ever be "over" when I have two foreign objects in my body for the rest of my life, seven scars, ongoing check-ups for 20 years, five years of Tamoxifen, and removal of my ovaries in two years, four months. Not sure where the "over" part comes in here.

I keep hanging onto the belief that through the rain I must go if, in the end, I want to find my rainbow, but it's hard when the rain continues to fall. It has indeed been one hell of a storm. The worst.

Wednesday, April 2, 2008
Frack, No Frick

I've been thinking about this whole upcoming procedure that I will be undergoing on May 6th. I have to be honest– I'm somewhat nervous about it, and I feel like I will be going right back to the crime scene...three days after the first anniversary of my mastectomy and five days before the Susan G. Komen Race for the Cure. It is all too familiar for me. I think this is probably as close to déjà vu as I might ever have been. I hope I don't have to get stabbed five times before they can actually get an IV in me this time and that I don't end up back in the ER the day after my release from the hospital...that would be creepy. While I have been rather anxious and easily distracted by my thoughts of the upcoming surgery, I have also been pondering some of the more significant issues at hand (or at boob, one might say).

As I have shared previously, Dr. Gimble, my plastic surgeon, will be removing a large portion of my back muscle (the latissimus muscle to be precise, which is the muscle under your shoulder blade that you work when you do pull-downs) and moving it to my chest area over the implant. In thinking about and trying to conceptualize all of this, I have come to realize that this means that I will have a "frack" (front/back). The following issues, concerns, and questions regarding my soon to be "frack" have been swirling around in my head:

1. When someone says they've got my back, it actually means they have my frack because if you got my back, then you have to have my front too because my back will soon be my front (Are you keeping up with this?).

2. What will be the appropriate way to wear backless shirts? Do I wear the opening in the back or the front or should I switch it around every fifteen minutes since half of my back will stay on my back and the other half will be on my front?

3. What happens if Dr. Gimbel accidentally moves my front to my back? Could this happen? Does that mean I would be somewhat backward?

4. What if someone tells me to give myself a "pat on the back?" Should I caress myself right there in front of the person? Eh...this actually wouldn't be any different from any other day. I touch the foobies all of the time, in front of pretty much anyone. And, I wonder why people are always staring at me. Here I thought it was my dashing good looks.

5. What will I do if a really handsome, super sexy fellow asks to give me a back massage? Oh BOY!

6. And last but not least– a frack should never be without a frick, right? But um, I don't have the appropriate anatomy to make myself a frick. It would add a whole new meaning to wearing dickies. That is funny, you know it is!

Truthfully, I don't think that any of this is funny, but my twisted sense of humor has been one of the very few things left intact through all of this cancer shit so I might as well use it.

Friday, April 4, 2008
National Young Adult Cancer Awareness Week

April 6-12 is National Young Adult Cancer Awareness Week. I'm hoping to use this week as an opportunity to educate others about cancer in young adults. We are a population that is under-represented in the cancer world (research, statistics, etc.), which is something I strive to change. It may not be today or tomorrow, but one day!

In celebration (not my word because I hardly think that the upcoming week is something to be celebrated), I will be attending the Pirate's game on Wednesday with some of my cancer cronies from the 20s-30s support group that I participate in at Gilda's Club. The tickets were donated to us by the players' wives. I will be sporting one of my many cancer shirts, of course!! I can't think of a better place to wear it to help increase awareness.

Friday, April 11, 2008
Pirates Game

On Wednesday, I went to the Pirates game with some of my cancer cronies from Gilda's Club. There were seven of us who went; six from the cancer support group and one supporter. The Pirates' wives gave us clubhouse seat tickets and Xavier Nagy and his wife donated $200 worth of voucher for food and beverages. I ate so much I thought I was going to combust.

It was a boring game (the Penguins were playing their first playoff game at that exact same time, so no one was there), but when you put six cancer survivors together in one place, you know it is going to be one heck of a good time regardless of the situation. We were laughing, hootin', and hollerin' the whole time. We did not stay for all fifteen innings but made it until the 10th or 11th. By the way, did you know that the Cubs have a player with the last name FUKUDOME (break it up—fuk u do me)? I've decided that I'm the President of his fan club.

This was the first outing we have had together as a group. It is so amazing to me how different we all are, but we have one thing that pulls us all together. It is the thing that has created such a strong bond between all of us. We know very little about one another, yet we feel like we have known each other for the longest time. These are the people that I feel like it is okay to cry in front of (and have) because they genuinely understand what it is that I'm going through. They give me inspiration and hope for a better tomorrow. They have become such important people in my life through an unfortunate set of circumstances.

I'm off to Florida on Sunday where I will be spending the week chillin' in the sun with my twelve layers of sunscreen, long sleeve shirt, and pants...no doubt, the guys will come running!!! I'm looking forward to a week of doing nothing and spending some quality time with my equally naughty friend, Amy.

Wednesday, April 23, 2008
Pre-operative Appointment

Yesterday, I went for my pre-operative appointment with my primary care physician, Dr. Gabriel Andrews, for my upcoming surgery on May 6th. I didn't have much time to sit in the waiting room to think before I was called back, which is a good thing. I sat in the patient room wearing my pretty, blue paper gown and white belt (who knew that paper gowns came with accessories) and waited for Dr. Andrews. As I sat there listening to my iPod, thoughts began swirling around in my head, and I could feel myself getting to the point of breaking down. I could feel my eyes welling up with tears at the thought of having to undergo another major surgery. When Dr. Andrews walked in, I think he was taken aback by my obvious distress. He didn't say much about that and asked questions about my health history (that seems funny to me...he is my doctor, he should know my health history) and current health (should know this too) and then examined my eyes, ears, throat, breathing, and abdominal area. He finally asked me how things are. I smiled as I always do and said, "It is what it is; I can't change it." He didn't have much to say to that, and honestly, I can't say I blame him...what do you say to that?

He left, and the nurse came in to draw some blood. I was still in tears at this time. Initially, she was planned on using a standard needle until I said that she needed to use a butterfly. She continued to comment about the size of my veins, so I knew that she wasn't going to get it. She was creeping me out because she put the needle in and then kept moving it around chasing the vein. Finally, she decided that someone else would need to come in to try. The second nurse came in and tried the right arm. She too thought that she would use a standard needle until I said that she should use the butterfly. She was successful. I sat there with my eyes closed, tears streaming down my face and my left arm over my head. The nurse was trying to comfort me the best she could and kept asking me if I was okay. I lied and said that I was fine. I got dressed, pulled myself together, and went out to the receptionist. She only looked at me and said, "Good luck with everything." The tears began to fall again.

I have come to realize I'm more anxious about this surgery than my mastectomy because everything was happening so fast last year that I didn't have time to think or process what was going on with me. I have had more time to digest what I'm currently going through. I would be lying if I said I'm not afraid...I'm scared as all hell. I get choked up and tear up every time I think about this surgery, and my stomach is so weak over all of this. The pain is excruciating, but I continue to tolerate it without any medication. I'm not sure I can explain this very well, but it is like someone is pulling the skin on the right side over to the left side and the left side over to the right side, which then makes it feel like someone is pulling the skin from my back around to the front. Gosh, do I hurt!!

Twelve days until surgery.

Thursday, April 24, 2008
Vacation!

I spent last week on vacation in Boynton Beach, Florida. While there, I met someone with whom I had an instant connection on so many different levels. He and I talked for many, many hours about life, death, love, happiness, and our situations (he does not have cancer). The day that we had to say goodbye was painful for both of us because we had a fantastic time together; it felt like I was leaving a long-time friend. What he said to me as we were parting ways rendered me speechless. He said, "You are the liveliest person that I have met in a very long time. You are amazing. Even with all that you have been through and are going through, you continue to smile and live life." I stood there not knowing what to say to this person that only spent a total of thirty hours with me but in that time could see something in me that I did not.

It was astonishing to me that much of what he and I spoke of was all that I have been thinking about over the past few months. I have been doing a lot of soul-searching and thinking about what is truly important in this life. Though I feel like I have lost a part of who I was before all of this, it is through that loss that I now realize that what I was living for previously is not what I should have been living for. I have come to learn that there is so much more to life, and I would much rather lead a meaningful life than to be wealthy. I know that everything happens for a reason and I whole-heartedly believe there is something much bigger I am meant to do with this experience than just getting through it; I do not think God brought me to this situation only to be a survivor. There is something much more meaningful that I am going to do with this. I have this feeling deep within my soul that somehow, in some way I'm going to use this experience to achieve the three goals I set for myself many, many years ago: Make a difference, change a life, and touch a heart. That will be the legacy that I leave behind.

I have had a poem on my office door for many years that gets to the heart of what I have been pondering lately.

How Do You Live Your Dash

I read of a man who stood to speak
At the funeral of a friend
He referred to the dates on her tombstone
From the beginning to the end.

He noted that first came her date of birth
And spoke the following date with tears,
But he said what mattered most of all

Was the dash between those years.

For that dash represents all the time
That she spent alive on Earth
And now only those who loved her
Know what that little line is worth.

For it matters not, how much we own;
The cars, the house, the cash,
What matters is how we live and love
And how we spend our dash.

So think about this long and hard,
Are there things you'd like to change?
For you never know how much time is left,
That can still be rearranged.

If we could just slow down enough
To consider what's true and real,
And always try to understand
The way other people feel.

And be less quick to anger,
And show appreciation more
And love the people in our lives
Like we've never loved before.

If we treat each other with respect,
And more often wear a smile
Remembering that this special dash
Might only last a little while.

So when your eulogy is being read
With your life's actions to rehash
Would you be proud of the things they say
About how you spent your dash?

-Author unknown

Sunday, April 27, 2008
Weekend Adventures

This weekend was the "kick-off" I needed right before my surgery. On Friday, I organized a happy hour with my cancer cronies. We went to the Pleasure Bar (not a strip club) in Bloomfield. There were seven of us plus my friend Annette. We had a great time watching the Pens game and happy hour ended up turning into happy hours by about five. Everyone had such a great time that they decided I need to organize all of our future happy hours. Oh, the pressure.

Saturday was uneventful. I had hoped to go skydiving but when I called Jeff at Skydive PA around 8:00 am, only seconds after I woke up from dreaming about skydiving. He didn't think the weather conditions would be suitable for a jump. Yeah, I'm thinking 55 mph winds would not be good. Jeff said that he would call me later in the day if things cleared up and he thought I could get a jump in, but if not, we planned for me to go first thing Sunday morning. I cleaned my apartment and did laundry in hopes of having things done before my surgery, so I won't be going crazy with not being able to do anything and having my place be a mess. My friend Nat called me later in the day. I met up with him and his family for dinner in Swissvale. It was a good time. Come to find out, one of the girls having dinner with us lives in the town right next to my hometown, and her last name is the same as one of the guys I used to hang out with all of the time in high school. Talk about a small world.

Today was a FABULOUS day!! I woke up at 7:30 am and anxiously waited for ten minutes to call Jeff to find out if he thought it would be a good day to jump. He was in the airplane when I called and said it was all a go. I hurriedly got a shower, ate some breakfast, made myself look pretty, and drove about 95 mph to Grove City. I was there by 9:20 am. I was so excited...I waited three hundred sixty-nine days and about nineteen hours to go skydiving again. This jump was different from my last tandem jump. Jeff was my tandem instructor for this jump, and we went up in a much smaller plane that only fits about five people, including the pilot. Last time, we scooted out to the edge of the plane, and I hung there at the mercy of the tandem instructor. This time, I held on to the inside of the plane, placed my foot on the platform outside of the plane, and when instructed, pushed off. It was awesome. We were "upside-down" for a few seconds before leveling off into a horizontal position. I was much more aware of things this time in comparison to last time– the wind, the speed, everything. The rush I felt this time was different from my previous jump as well. Though it was still a huge adrenaline rush, I think that my next jump needs to be a solo jump to get the thrill that I am seeking. Jeff let me control the chute for a little bit, and we hung out in the sky for a while, which was super cool. We were gliding along in the spring breeze. I got my jump logbook and the class list for the solo jump training. Jeff and

John (my tandem instructor from last year) seem to think that I should get licensed and told me I would really fit in with everyone. In talking to one of the guys, I found out that there is a "jump for the cure" to benefit breast cancer. How awesome is that? Now I definitely have to train to jump solo!

After leaving Grove City, I drove to Monaca to meet up with Denny. He is a friend of a friend that calls me anytime there is a motorcycle ride to see if I want to go. I hadn't been able to go until today. I thought about not going for maybe a millisecond because I have a report that I need to get done for work. Motorcycle ride or writing a report. Hmm, let's see...motorcycle ride!! I'm so glad that I ended up going because it was a great time. We rode to Saxonburg and had lunch at Rowe's. It was so nice to be on the back of a bike with the wind blowing through my hair and the sound and smell of motorcycle exhaust all around me. I chilled back there thinking about how precious life is and how I don't ever want to let an opportunity to enjoy life pass me by. It was a very tranquil feeling. We rode for about three or four hours. They all laughed at me when I told them that I was going to go home and smell myself. I love the smell of motorcycle exhaust. I swear if I could only bottle this up!!

I have the biggest smile on my face, and I feel like the weight of the world has been lifted off of my shoulders! What a great way to head into the week before my surgery.

Tuesday, May 6, 2008
Surgery #4

Well, here it is...the day of my fourth surgery. *vomit*

I have to be at the hospital at 5:15 am for surgery at 7:30 am. I will be sporting the new t-shirt that I purchased for my surgery. It says, "Cancer Can Kiss My Ass." I will be meeting my parents and my Grammy at the hospital. I realize that might seem odd, but that is my choice as I don't do well with someone in my apartment with me the night before my surgery. I need the time alone to reflect on things.

I'm pretty anxious right now. It is after 12:00 am, and I'm still awake. One would think that I might be in bed trying to rest the night before a big surgery, but I can't seem to let my mind or body relax enough to even think about crawling in bed. My stomach is upset right now to the point of needing or wanting to vomit. I have about a thousand thoughts running through my head at warp speed. Though all of the circumstances surrounding this surgery are eerily similar to my surgery last year at this time, I am much more aware of what is going on around and within me. I have had too much time to think about what is going on this time in comparison to last year when everything was pretty much a big blur. It is all very unsettling to me and though I have been told several times to "try to not think about it," I can only say that would be like asking the Pope not to pray– not going to happen.

On a positive note, I found out that my story will hopefully be published in the Pittsburgh Post-Gazette on Thursday. It will be either on the front page or in the local news section. The photographers will be coming into the hospital on Wednesday for a photoshoot. I decided to get all decked out for them and wear a beautiful, repeatedly recycled hospital gown...opening in the front, of course. We discussed staging a photograph for the article, but I had proposed doing it while I'm in the hospital. I want people to see the real, raw, in your face side of this disease and not a pretty young lady that no one would ever guess had cancer. Since it will run on the day of my hospital release, I have my doubts that I will get it unless I steal the paper from someone in my apartment building. (I would never!!!)

Tuesday, May 6, 2008
Written by my BFF, Ken

The day of surgery #4 is here. Melissa was at the hospital by 5:15 am for the 7:30 surgery. The first text (at least the one I received) was at 5:16 am. Our princess was true to form on that. All it took was a few simple words, "I am ready to vomit!" That pretty much summed it up.

Melissa's mom called around 11:30 am with an update that the four hours of surgery went well. The surgeon had good reports, but it was still off to the recovery room for our favorite survivor! After a long stay in recovery (she handles the drug thing so well), she was back in her room.

At 4:10 pm she sounded really groggy and still half-kicked. She was pretty spent as well but she still had her sense of humor. I felt bad making her laugh. Even through the chemicals, she is still feeling pain.

At any rate, she is doing well but will need the time to get her feet back under her.

I know she thanks you for keeping her in your thoughts and prayers!

God bless Sweet Melissa!

Thursday, May 8, 2008
Written by my BFF, Ken

It is now two days after surgery and Melissa is hanging in there. She is sounding more and more like herself... at least in between the waves of nausea that seem to be hitting her. She was able to eat some carrot cake last night, which made her very happy.

Because of the surgery, it is very difficult for her to move her right arm. She is still in quite a bit of pain, but she is toughing it out. The doctor is scheduled to see her this morning at 7:30 am to take a look at how she is healing and make the call as to whether or not she can be released from the hospital.

She continues to thank everyone for the prayers and thoughtfulness. She is anxious to be home in her place that is more comfortable, but she will still need a few extra hands here and there to help her along. I know we are all out there for her!

Friday, May 9, 2008
Written by my BFF, Ken

Melissa is now home although continues to be less than comfortable given the nausea. Vicodin doesn't treat her very well. She is doing her best to rest easy, but that too comes and goes. She sounds more and more herself, but you can tell she is still a little guarded at times. The little things like laughing and sneezing are excruciating to her.

The good news is her being home AND that the wheelchair is getting primed for her second shot at the Race for the Cure on Mother's Day. It will be a repeat performance being wheeled through the course, although the driver on the #6 chair will be different, sorry to say. But she is in great hands. She is looking forward to it, but she is looking forward to breaking the wheelchair streak next year when she WILL walk under her own power!

Keep thinking of her, as I know you will!

Wednesday, May 14, 2008
May 6, 2007- Surgery #4

I awoke at 3:30 am after going to bed at 1:00 am. My stomach was uneasy, and my mind started going a thousand mph. A single tear fell from the eye and before any more could fall; I said to myself, "Melissa, you can't do this right now." I got out of bed, showered, and got ready for my big day. I arrived at UPMC Shadyside at 5:05 am. I walked for what seemed like five-hundred miles to the Family Surgical Lounge and checked in with the receptionist. She made me feel bad that my family was not there yet, so I called my parents to see where there were; they were on their way. A group of about ten of us were taken upstairs to pre-op at 5:15 am. I got undressed and sat in my room anxiously waiting for someone to get me all geared up for surgery. I sent a simple text message to Ken that said, "I'm ready to vomit." We were only able to exchange a few texts before I got yelled at by the nurse because the cardiac unit was next door. Hello...how would I know this?

I called my parents again. They were downstairs waiting to come to pre-op. Before they arrived, the nurse came to put my IV in my left arm. I recommended that she use a heated compress to help get a vein. At first, she didn't seem to think that was necessary but then realized that I knew what I was talking about. She was able to get the IV in on the first try, thank goodness. Then she realized that I had make-up on and about freaked. She made me wipe it off because I might get a corneal abrasion from sleeping with my make-up on. Newsflash, I wore make-up during all three of my other surgeries. When my parents and Grammy arrived, it looked like I had been crying because my make-up was smeared down my face. Before they came into the room, I had to use the two moist cloths the nurse had given me to wipe down my chest, arms, and legs. I'm not sure what was in them, but my legs started to itch, and I developed a rash. The nurse told me not to scratch or rub them...easy for her to say when she isn't the one having the reaction. Another nurse then came in and said that she needed to take some more blood. I'm still not sure why even though I do remember asking her. She tried on the left side without any luck. She was hesitant to use the right side because there was a sign above my head indicating the right side couldn't be used. The nurse was about to stab me again when Dr. Gimbel walked in and asked her what she was doing. He told her that I did not need any blood drawn. I mouthed "thank you" to him. My family left the room, and he made pretty pictures on my chest and back. A short time later, I was taken off to surgery. I was more emotional this time than previously and was crying as I was taken away from my parents. I only remember being wheeled into the OR and taking in four deep breaths. I was out.

The surgery took approximately three and a half to four hours. I was in recovery by 11-11:30 am. The nurse attempted to wake me up but only did so for a few seconds– long enough for me to feel them pulling the breathing tube out of my throat, and then I was out again. I was in recovery until about 3:30 pm. The nurse tried to wake me numerous times, but I was having no part of that. The only time I wanted anything to do with her was when my mouth was dry. At some point during my stay in recovery, she took her lunch break. I became distraught when I realized that she was gone and nobody else seemed to be concerned with me. I watched a nurse walk by me numerous times, but she never stopped. It took all of my energy to ask her if I could have something to drink, which was denied.

I was so relieved to see my nurse come back from lunch a few minutes later. Upon her return, she wanted to empty out my drains. When she moved my right arm, I let out the loudest squeal because of the pain. She apologized profusely. After a few more hours of trying to rouse me, it was time to go to my room. When the transporters came to take me to my room, I remember the nurse telling them to be very careful with my right side because I was in significant pain. My parents and Grammy were in my room before I arrived but were asked to leave while I was transferred from the gurney to the bed. There were three of them moving me; one down by my feet, one up by my head, and one on my right side. Unlike at Magee, I wasn't asked to move myself from the gurney to the bed. Instead, the two girls at both ends picked up the draw sheet and the nurse on my right SHOVED me. I'm not over exaggerating this...she pushed with a lot of force on my right side. I screamed from the pain and began crying. I wanted nothing more at that moment then to grab her by her hair and punch her in the face (and I'm not a violent person). My pain was now magnified by 10. I then discovered that I didn't have a catheter or a morphine drip. Talk about cruel and usual punishment. I wasn't very engaging with my family because the pain from this surgery was so much worse than the bilateral mastectomy. There was no laughing and joking around. I lay there silently wishing for the pain to stop and wonder why I have to endure all of this. If I spoke with anyone that evening, I don't remember at all. My dad and Grammy stayed until sometime in the evening, but my mom spent the night with me.

Thursday, May 15, 2008
Hospital Stay

I didn't have a good night on Tuesday at all. My mom stayed the night with me on Tuesday, but I was unable to sleep because of her snoring. I spent most of the morning hours text messaging Justin...thank goodness he lives in a different time zone and is a night owl.

Since I had saline being pushed through my IV, I had to use the bathroom frequently. The nurse and aide seemed to be annoyed every time I had to use the bathroom. Neither of them was much help to get me out of or back in bed. The nurse became agitated with me when I repeatedly asked her about my Tamoxifen. Finally, she gave it to me at about 10:00 pm and acted as though that was my usual time to take it so I certainly shouldn't have had my panties in a bunch (okay, I wasn't wearing any). She returned to give me another shot to help prevent blood clots. I explained that I already had a shot so I didn't think I should get another. It almost worked, but she came back a few minutes later and said I would be getting two a day in the abdomen. I had never gotten a shot in my abs before, so I was naturally a bit nervous, plus I hate needles. Thinking that she was going to be gentle with me and not really having any other option anyway, I lay there at her mercy. She grabbed me by the skin on my abdomen and stabbed me like she was taking a knife to her worst enemy. I was completely shocked. My experience with the hospital up to this point was not a positive one, and I was beginning to get pissed off at myself for not pushing Dr. Gimbel, my plastic surgeon, to do the surgery at Magee.

When morning came, I was so excited that I would be getting a new nurse but then to my surprise, my night nurse walked in. UGH! She was still there. I pretended like I cared that she worked long hours and asked her about her shift. I was trying to find out if she would be returning to work that evening, and thankfully, she was not. Woo Hoo. Wednesday was rather uneventful in the hospital. Dr. Gimbel came to check on me and suggested I stay another night. Boo! I briefly expressed my painful experience with the transporters and the night nurses. I asked to be switched to Vicodin because the Percocet wasn't doing anything to control the pain and when they pushed morphine through my IV, I wanted to jump right out of my skin from the pain. I got cleaned up, took a walk, and then had my photoshoot for the Pittsburgh Post-Gazette. I got lots of phone calls, but the one that sticks out most in my head is that from my Uncle Warren. We spoke for maybe a minute and a half before he broke down into tears and had to get off the phone. It tore me apart. My dad and brother came to visit, then my Uncle Dave showed up. They stayed until about 2:00 pm. My friend Annette came to visit in the evening. I asked her to take me for another walk. We sat around chatting; she helped me to get my things ready for discharge the next day and then had to leave. My night nurse and nurse's aide were so sweet and helpful on Wednesday night. They didn't become agitated with me and were gentle when I had to get the shot. I actually slept through some of the night on Wednesday.

Dr. Gimbel woke me up on Thursday morning. He checked my incisions and drains. He was pleased with how things were healing and said that I could be discharged. I was initially okay with this, but then I started getting sick and was nervous about being sent home. My breakfast was delivered at approximately 8 am, but I could only eat some of it. About ten minutes later, I started to vomit. I called the nurse for some anti-nausea medicine. I managed to find a way to lie on my left side and didn't move for hours on end because every time I moved, I felt like I was going to throw up. I got sick two more times before my dad came at about 12:15 pm.

My lunch was delivered by a sweet, young guy that had a horrified look on his face when he saw me. He looked like he was about to break down into tears. He asked me if there was anything that he could do for me, but I assured him that there was not. I managed to sit up after a few minutes and ate only the mashed potatoes. My dad helped me get my clothes and bag into the bathroom so I could get cleaned up and ready for discharge. I waited for about 10 minutes for a transporter to take me to the car. I took the vomit container with me because my stomach was still weak. We got on the elevator, and of course, it stopped on every floor. I thought for sure I was going to get sick every time the elevator dropped. The girl kept asking me if I was okay, but I couldn't say anything for fear that if I did, that would be the point when I would start vomiting.

The whole way home, I sat with my head in the vomit container. My dad got me settled in and went to the store to get my prescriptions and some food. I ate some crackers and drank some ginger ale in hopes of settling my stomach. My friend Annette stopped by to visit and gave me the information I needed to go to Philip Pelusi to get my hair washed since my right arm is nonfunctional at this point. I started to feel weak in my stomach again and sat for several minutes with my head in the vomit container. I laughed while telling Annette and my dad that this was a perfect Kodak moment and that I was having performance anxiety but that I would freely vomit as soon as Annette was gone. Sure enough, I vomited about five minutes after she was gone. Not only was the vomiting painful, but I was left in excruciating pain all day because I was throwing up the Vicodin.

My dad stayed the night with me, but I wasn't able to get any sleep because he snores, too!!

Friday, May 16, 2008
What I See

Friday, May 9th, was the first day that I was able to shower on my own, meaning that I would have to take off the surgical bra and dressings. As I've not had positive experiences with this in the past, I didn't know if I was ready to see what they had done to me this time. I stood in front of my bathroom mirror with nothing on but the surgical bra. As many times as I tried, I couldn't bring myself to look and stepped outside of view from the mirror before removing everything. Eh, I figured I could try again tomorrow. Saturday and Sunday came and went, but I still couldn't bring myself to stand in front of the mirror as I took off the surgical bra. Finally, on Monday, I decided that I needed to look. I forced myself to stand there while I removed the surgical bra and dressings. I stood there in awe, taking in all that my body had endured. I had expected to have three incisions and one JP drain (boobie tubies, as I like to call them). When Dr. Gimbel and I spoke, he said that he would be making a new incision under the right implant, but that apparently didn't work out for him. I have one incision on my left side as he replaced the smaller implant with the one that was supposed to be placed in there. I have two incisions on the right side; one is along the same incision line as the mastectomy and the insertion of the implant, which runs diagonally down the middle and the other incision runs along the upper quarter of the foobie area. The incisions come together at the ends, making a football-like shape.

Hmm....so it would seem that the scar will be visible to others if I wear something like a tank top. I don't like that much at all. The shape of the right side is distorted, and it looks like a deflated ball. After a few minutes of staring at myself, I turn to the side to look at the drain sites. Ew.... I had to turn away immediately. They were so nasty. When I felt ready to look again, I turned to the side and took that in. I have one coming from the front that runs up into my armpit and one coming from my back. The tubes are much larger than what I had last time, and I could see that my skin wasn't stitched up around the tubes. At this point, I thought I had seen all that I could see. I didn't want to see anymore, but I only had one more to look at, so why stop now? How traumatizing could it be? I went into my bedroom and turned around in front of the full-length mirror to see the incision on my back. Eek!! What little I saw was not pleasing to my peepers. I turned away and stood there not knowing what to do.

I knew there was no way I could see the entire length of the incision by looking in the mirror. So, I grabbed my camera and took a picture of it. The first one I took didn't look too bad. Then I had the great idea of standing backward in the mirror and taking the picture. Holy Hell, Batman!! It was so much bigger than I had expected. I knew that it was going to be big, but not that big. It runs from near my spine diagonally down to my side. I continued to stand there looking at all of what I had been through...wow, is it possible that one person could endure so much all at once? With my new incisions and the drains, I will now have nine scars; seven on the right side and two on the left side. But I know that these scars are the easy ones; they will heal in a few weeks. The hardest scars to heal are the ones on my heart, my self-esteem, my self-image, and my soul. There aren't enough band-aids, gauze, or medical tape in this world to bandage up those scars. They run deep and bleed heavily.

On Wednesday, May 14th, I went to my first follow-up appointment with Dr. Gimbel. I'm happy to say that this appointment makes the 3rd that I have gotten through without crying. Woo Hoo. He checked the incisions and is pleased with how they are healing. He is a bit concerned with the reddish color of the right side, and on top of that, I have been running a low-grade fever for a few days. He considered leaving the boobie tubies but ultimately decided that they could be removed. It was much more painful than my last experience. Though I'm numb under my armpit and on the right side of my chest and back, I could feel when he undid the stitches and pulled the drains out. When he took the one out from my back, it felt like he squirted water up the inside of my back. It was the craziest feeling. He left the steri-strips on; they supposedly will fall off on their own. When the nurse was helping me to get my dressings and bra back on, she asked me if I wanted all that dressing in my bra. I simply said, "Yes, it's the only thing that makes me look even." She left the office in a hurry.

Dr. Gimbel recommended that I start wearing a sports bra with some back support. He suggested that I come back in two weeks and, at that time, he hopes that we can start the expansion of the right side. When I asked him if the right side would look like the left side, to my complete devastation, he said that it will never look like the left side again no matter how hard he tries. Great. Just great. The nurse came back in with a book for post-mastectomy prosthesis. I wasn't prepared for that and hadn't even thought about it, but considering that I have two weddings this summer, I need to do something to even myself out.

So here it is, Friday, May 16th, and it's been ten days since my surgery. I've decided to stop taking the Vicodin and suck up the pain (because I'm stubborn), which at times is more than I think I can handle. I ordered my prosthesis last night, but I'm not sure how I feel about it. As if all that I have been through isn't enough, now I have to wear a prosthesis. Crap! I tried sleeping in my bed last night instead of on the chaise lounge, but I tossed and turned all night. The problem is that I can't sleep on my stomach, I can't sleep on my right side, and I can't have the right side of my back flat on the bed, so my sleeping positions are limited. UGH! My range of motion sucks on the right side, and I have limited strength in my arm. The left side isn't all that much better. I got up this morning and cried because I'm so tired of all cancer has done and continues to do to me. I'm tired of having to be strong and holding myself up all the time. I'm tired of being poked, prodded, stabbed, ripped apart, and sewn back together. I'm sick and tired of being sick and tired!

I HATE CANCER!!!!!!!!!!

Monday, May 19, 2008
When Life Leads You Where You Don't Want to Go

For all of us, to varying degrees, life takes us in a direction we may have never wanted to go. We all think that we have so much control over our own destiny but do we really? We spend so much of our time planning out our lives that we often forget how to live our lives. I can tell you that if I had control over my own destiny, it most certainly wouldn't have ever involved cancer. Somehow when I was working out my five- and ten-year plans, I didn't take into consideration the fact that I would have cancer at the age of 31. It didn't fit into the top five things that I wanted to achieve in this life: 1) Be successful in my career, 2) Purchase another house, 3) Travel the world, 4) Fall in love with someone who is absolutely head-over-heels crazy for me, and 5) Have children: twins - a boy (Trenton) and a girl (Ellie); in that order. I was part of the rat race that we call life– looking to do better than the next person, looking to get more things, and looking out for only myself. It is no wonder that cancer has left me falling end over end at the speed of light.

My life most certainly has not led me where I wanted to go, and I sit for hours and hours contemplating the reasons and what it all means for me. I'm not sure I'm even close to figuring it out. I'm not sure that I ever will. I have been robbed of so many things for reasons that I will never understand. I don't know where life is taking me, but I often think about where I might go "after" all of this. I wonder if I will get through this and find my happiness again. Will I stay where I am? Will I fall in love? Will I change someone's life by sharing my experience? Will I hold the hand of another young cancer patient as she/he travels through her/his cancer journey? Will my words inspire another? Will I be the source of strength for someone else who has hit rock bottom? Or will I fight and fight, only to end up losing the battle in the end anyway? I don't know the answers, and I'm not sure that I would want to know. The reality is that any of those could be the answer. They could all be the answer.

Obviously, after having been knocked on my ass by cancer, I've been left trying to pick up the pieces of my life. I feel like I'm sitting at a crossroads that goes in five different directions with not a clue as to which one I should choose. I have not yet managed to stand steady on my feet, but I figure it's like a baby learning to walk. I'm going to get up and fall back down a few times before I get the hang of this again. It's going to be a long road ahead to rebuild my life, and I'm going to have to learn to live with this cancer thing. One thing I know for sure is that whether I'm still sitting down or running full speed ahead, I'm not going to let life pass me by. I'm not going to waste my time trying to control my own destiny; I've learned it's out of my hands anyway. I'm not sure who it was that said you only get one chance in this life, but I would safely assume that he/she didn't have a date with death. I've danced with death, and I'm so grateful to have been given a second chance. I have given up trying to plan out the next five or 10 years and have learned to simply live for today. I will worry about tomorrow when it comes.

I still want to be successful in my career, but I no longer think that the more I'm paid, the more successful I am. I have a completely different view of measuring my success. While I would love to travel the world and take in all the beauty and wonders of it, I have decided that I want to visit with friends and family instead. Whether I admit it or not, I have someone who is head-over-heels crazy about me, but I've been too busy pushing him away for fear of rejection. He is persistent, though, and hasn't gone anywhere.

I don't necessarily like the direction that life has taken me, but I'm ready to get back up on my feet and start down another path to see what this crazy thing called life has in store for me next. It truly is about learning how to dance in the rain!!!

Tuesday, May 20, 2008
Baby Steps to Normalcy

As you can probably imagine, this surgery has left me dysfunctional in a lot of ways. I hadn't been able to wash my own hair and was going to Philip Pelusi to have them wash and braid it. I finally washed my hair on Saturday. It took me about four hours, and I was worn out by the end of it, but I did it! I drove myself to church on Sunday even though I have limited range of motion on my right side. I will admit that I was scared out of my mind, but I made it there and back safely. On Monday, I finally braved the shower. I had been taking baths up to this point because the water pressure of my shower would be like standing under the Niagara Falls. I learned my lesson from my previous surgery. I about jumped out of my skin when the water hit me in the back, but I was able to manage. I finally slept in my bed last night. I figured out a way to lie on my stomach or back without any of the incisions touching the bed, which made me happy. I still struggle with changing positions because I can't put weight on my right arm, and I can't use it to pull myself up. Getting myself out of bed is quite the task, but at least I was able to get some good sleep.

We all take the simple things in life (showering, driving, getting out of bed without any effort, etc.) for granted but when it is taken away (even if temporarily), you gain greater value for being able to do them. It most certainly provides a perspective into the lives of those who struggle with these mundane tasks each and every day.

And today, I'm doing my part in preventing forest fires– I'm going to shave my legs!!!!

Wednesday, May 21, 2008
WHY?

I have come to realize that throughout this experience I have not asked, "Why me?" It was not something that I really took the time to think about. I kind of started pondering that question as I sat on my couch this evening in rather excruciating pain. Before I would let my mind wander too far with that question, I sent a text message to my friend Kyle who has multiple sclerosis and has recently had another episode with it. He is someone very special to me because we share a bond that is much different than that of my other pre-cancer friends. He is a source of strength and an inspiration to me. I was taken aback when he indicated that he is not doing well and that he will be spending the next ten days in the hospital undergoing a new treatment. Then it hit me like a ton of bricks...Why Me? Why Him? Why Any of Us? I don't understand it at all.

Okay, so we all know that I apparently got the wrong biological sperm donor, but that doesn't make it any easier to understand. Here I am at the age of 32, and I have been hacked apart more times in the past year than I care to even recount at this point. A part of my femininity has been stolen from me. All of what I have left that makes me female will be taken in two years (well, that's the doctor's plan anyway). I have been robbed of my dreams to one day have my own children and leave a legacy behind in them. I have been deeply scarred- mentally and emotionally. All this, while the person (I refuse to call him a man) who I inherited this mutated gene from continues to live his life– a cancer-free life at that. How is it that someone who attempted to take two small children away from their mother against their will, putting them in harm's way, attempted to cause harm to their mother, and then ultimately walked away from them without even a glance back manages to go through life on Easy Street? It makes no sense to me at all. What makes me deserve this and not him?

Every time I think about where this disease came from, it's like someone taking a knife and stabbing me repeatedly in the heart. I didn't turn my back on him. When I was young and didn't know better, I wanted him to be a part of my life. I remember being a young girl, maybe four years old, sitting on my front porch for hours waiting for the biological sperm donor to come to get me while all of my friends and my brother played. You know what? He never came, and I was crushed. I remember going to his house once and hated it because his wife wouldn't let me eat my spaghetti until I held my fork correctly. I remember telling him that I wanted twin Cabbage Patch dolls for Christmas one year. Well, I don't know what it was that I got that year, if anything at all, but what I do know is his wife got twin Cabbage Patch dolls. Those are the only memories I have of him because I figured things out quickly and came to realize that this person wasn't anyone I wanted in my life. He made some half-hearted attempts a handful of times after that, but I wanted nothing to do with

135

him. I realized at a young age that my dad had been where he always was, right there beside me...tucking me in at night, playing jacks with me, wiping the tears from my eyes when I fell, teaching me right from wrong, and loving me the way only a real father can. But it is still a devastating blow knowing that the cowardly sperm donor has caused me the most excruciating pain I have ever experienced in my life, which has resulted in the scars that I will carry on the outside and the inside for the rest of my life. As if the blows I had taken as a small child weren't bad enough, how do I wrap my mind around all of that without questioning why me?

And there is my sweet Kyle. He is only 25 years old and has been dealing with the MS for a few years now. There are days when he can't walk or see. Sometimes he has to use a cane, and the doctors tell him that he will be in a wheelchair soon; they are surprised he is not already. There are days when he tells me that his legs feel like they are on fire. I don't understand why he has been dealt this hand. He is one of the sweetest and most genuine guys I know. I think he may be one of the very few good guys left out there. I've seen the love that he has for his family and friends. He is like I am in that we both care deeply for those we love and will do anything to protect them (that comes from both of us being a cancer- the zodiac sign, not the disease). I don't understand "why Kyle" when I look at some others who have less character and value for themselves and others.

There are so many others going through things that I can't and don't understand. I have a hard time wrapping my mind around my dealing with cancer and Kyle's dealing with the MS but most of all I can't even begin to fathom an innocent baby that hasn't even been given a chance at life without having to fight every single day. WHY??????

I don't know why we are chosen to go through the trials and tribulations that we do, nor do I intend to sit around trying to figure it out, but I needed to get that off my chest.

Wednesday, May 28, 2008
BP (Boobie Pumping) Station

Well, today was my first trip back to the BP (boobie pumping) station, also known as my plastic surgeon's office, for (re)expansion number one. I went by myself since I've almost mastered one-handed driving. I didn't have to sit for more than a minute in the waiting room before Judy, the nurse, took me back. I laid down with my iPod in my ears while listening to my cancer comfort songs and shaking my legs like I always do when I'm nervous as I waited for Dr. Gimbel, my plastic surgeon. He checked all of my incisions and felt it was time to remove all of the steri-strips. I had to cover my ears because the sound of him ripping them off made me cringe. I was a bit nervous about him taking the one off my back and the one on the upper part of the foobie because I have the most pain in those two areas. He asked me several times if I wanted to take them off...NO THANK YOU! He is pleased with how all of the incisions have healed and was happy to see that I have not had any more drainage since the JP drains were taken out.

This was the first time that I have seen my incisions without the steri-strips on them and should have known better than to look down. The football-shaped incision on my right side looked worse with the steri-strips off. I almost broke down into tears but was able to maintain my composure. I only said, "Ew, that's so gross." He thought I was referencing all of the dried blood, but that wasn't it at all. The issue is that the right side has an indentation and is hollow on the upper left corner whereas the left implant is even and full the entire way around. I asked him if the hollow portion would eventually fill out and he said that it probably will not because of all the damage caused by the radiation and the manipulation of skin, muscle, and tissue that has occurred on the right side. He said the objective is to make me look as symmetrical as possible in clothing and of course, me being who I am, I reminded him that tank tops are clothing as well. Unfortunately, he seems to think that when all is said and done with this, I will not look symmetrical in tank tops. UGH!

I also asked him about the discoloration of my skin and the different texture from one area to the next. He indicated that this is due to the impact of the radiation. The right side is blotchy and red under the implant and tight; the middle, where the football shape is, continues to be white and tender like the real me used to be; the upper left corner is a yellowish-red, wrinkly, and has an odd feeling to it. I think maybe I will get the Steelers emblem tattooed there since I already have the red and yellow and I have a football in the middle of the right side.

After he answered what I am sure felt like five-thousand questions, including explaining what they did with my arm during the surgery (They stacked it up with pillows. I had a mental image of them dropping down a strap from the ceiling and wrapping it around my wrist), he filled me up with 75cc of saline. He seems to think that I won't have the muscle spasms that I experienced last year, which would be a positive thing. I told him that it was pure hell the night before I was able to get the muscle relaxers. He smiled and said that he remembers where he was when I called him, so I'm thinking I left a lasting impression. He wants me to call him if I start having the muscle spasms again so he can call in the prescription. I'm crossing my fingers and tootsies that I don't need them this time. He thinks I will need to have two or three more expansions, which will occur every two weeks instead of every week and a half like last year. I'm still not permitted to lift more than three pounds on my right side. I'm not allowed to do anything that would cause strain on my back for the next month.

I told him my range of motion is terrible, despite my doing the wall climbs at least three times per day. He asked me to raise my right arm and said that I need to start physical therapy as soon as possible, so he wrote a script for eight weeks of physical therapy. Boo!!! I was so hoping I wouldn't ever have to do that again either but apparently, I don't know how to take the "easy" road. I think my cancer motto should be "GO BIG OR GO HOME!" I go back for my next fill up at the BP station on June 11th, and then I see my medical oncologist on June 12th. All these appointments make it feel like "old times" (okay, maybe only like a year ago "old times"). I'm feeling so nostalgic right now.

Tuesday, June 3, 2008
Things Could be Worse????

Throughout our lives, each one of us faces a different set of circumstances, trials, and tribulations. While society views some things as being worse than others, we all have things that we have to deal with, no matter how "big" or "small." I've come to hate the expression, "It could be worse." I can't even begin to count how many different times I have had someone tell me that things could be worse. Though I know that it is said with all good intentions, it most certainly doesn't make me feel any better. I'm sure it is easy for anyone outside of my circumstance to think that those words might provide me with some comfort, but they don't. Not at all. Honestly, it makes me feel as though all that I have been through is being minimized.

I can only imagine that most people tell me that things could be worse because I am still alive while others have lost their battle. Outside of that, I'm not sure how anyone thinks that fighting cancer could be worse. While I'm grateful that I am still here among the living, I will be candid and say that I have days when I think it would be so much easier if I weren't. Sometimes I get so tired of waking up day in and day out and having to deal with all of this. There are days when I want to throw my hands up in the air, wave the white surrender flag, and say, "Okay cancer, you win."

Every single day is a struggle from the moment I wake up in the morning until the time that I go to sleep, if that even happens. Every single day, I wake up and carry the weight of the world on my shoulders. I wake up every day and see the scars and the damage left behind from cancer. I wake up every day knowing that at any given moment my body could betray me again. I wake up every day knowing that my hopes and dreams have been shattered. I wake up every day knowing that my life has been turned upside down because of the mutated gene passed on from someone that never cared if I were dead or alive. I wake up every day prepping myself to make those around me think that everything is fine, even when it is not. I wake up every day wishing that things could be normal again and dealing with the emotional scars. I wake up every day worrying about how distorted I might look to others. I wake up every day and force myself to push back my thoughts and emotions so that I can function throughout the day. I wake up every day hating myself and all that I have been through and all that I have yet to go through. Really? Things could be worse?

I know that it is hard to understand something that someone has never experienced personally, but that is probably all the more reason not to say, "Things could be worse."

Thursday, June 5, 2008
Physical Therapy

I started physical therapy on Tuesday. The appointment took about an hour and a half to two hours. The physical therapist had to check my range of motion and my strength. I already knew that my left side has some minor limitations, but the right side is very limited, and I have no strength in my right arm. She had me do some exercises with a cane. I put my left hand at the bottom of the cane and my right hand at the top and then pushed straight up as far as I could get my right arm to my ear. Then I pushed out to the side. The physical therapist then did some stretching exercises with me where she pushed my right arm straight up and then out to the side. Apparently, my face tells it all because she knew I was in pain before I even had to tell her.

I was pretty sore when we were finished. I iced my shoulder and back as soon as I got home and popped some Tylenol too, so you know I was in pain. It continued to get worse as the evening progressed, and I woke up super stiff on Wednesday morning. I took it easy throughout most of the day on Wednesday and did my PT exercises while watching the Penguins game. I iced it again. The swelling/inflammation seemed to go down some.

I returned for my second physical therapy session today. I had to do my exercises with the cane, and then they added five new ones (holy crap, Batman!!!!). I had to sit in a chair with my arm on the bed and stretch it straight out in front of me while I tried to lean forward as far as I could. I then had to switch to the side. Then she had me put my elbow at a 90-degree angle, rest it on the bed, and lean forward as far as I could. Let me tell you how much I hate this exercise. It is an exercise that focuses on your pectoral muscles, and when you have had your pecs removed, it makes this exercise not so fun. I would seriously rather dig my eyes out with pencils than have to do that specific exercise. They made me do the same one last year except that I was standing in a corner with my arms at a 90-degree angle against the wall and had to push forward. Um yeah, it sucks. Anyway, I digress.

The other two exercises were with the pulley. I had to alternate back and forth with my right and left arms to the front and then again to the side. Honestly, I was about done with all of this PT stuff after the fourth exercise, so by the time I actually finished, I was ready to go back to bed. My physical therapist then stretched my right arm out by lifting it straight up, out to the side, and up at an angle (pushing the inner part of my elbow toward my head). My back and side under my arm are swollen and inflamed again. I will be icing it throughout the evening, but if the pain doesn't subside, I will resort to the Vicodin! Did I mention that I LOVE physical therapy??

140

I also wanted to clarify that my last entry wasn't intended to hurt anyone's feelings or upset anyone, but I felt like I needed to be honest in that I find no comfort in being told that things could be worse. I'm not offended or hurt when I'm told that, I can't handle hearing it right now. This is so hard for me to deal with, and most people will never know the full extent of my pain because I try not to let it show. Just when I thought I was getting to a little bit of a better place with all of this, it has sucked me right back down. The physical damage that has been left behind from the radiation and the last surgery on my right side has handed me a blow to my self-image and my self-esteem. There are days when I wish that I had the nerve to show everyone what I'm dealing with, but I can't bring myself to show anyone. I'm a complete mess, on the inside and out.

Friday, June 6, 2008
Facing My Demons

I knew that eventually, I would come face-to-face with the sperm donor (my biological father) who is responsible for passing along his faulty DNA to me, but I had hoped it wouldn't be so soon in my journey. Tomorrow is my cousin Dina's wedding. Unfortunately, the sperm donor and his wicked wife will be there. I'm starting to get nervous and somewhat sick to my stomach over this. Initially, I had a date but found out a few hours ago that he is unable to go. That is a whole other issue that I will deal with later. Now I have to go and do this on my own. *vomit*

I'm not sure that I even want to go at this point, but it would break my cousin's heart if I didn't show up and I couldn't do that to her. I know that this is her day, and I won't do anything to ruin it or take that away from her, but I also know that I'm emotionally not ready to face this demon.

I have so much anger inside of me that I only hope and pray that, should he approach me, I handle myself with grace and kindly ask that he not speak to me. I have so much to say to him and yet, nothing to say to him. My mom always taught me that if I don't have anything nice to say, don't say anything at all. Well, this would be the perfect example of when I need to listen to my mother. Since my cousin Dennis will be going, I will be hanging out with him instead. Thank goodness for him!

Wednesday, June 11, 2008
Taking the High Road

Saturday was Dina's wedding, and it was the first time that I came face-to-face with the sperm donor that passed along the genetic mutation, as well as his family that I don't have any contact with outside of my Uncle Dave, Aunt Shirley, and my cousin Dennis. My cousin Dennis and I rode together to the wedding. When we got into the church, I stood for a while checking out the scene. Beth (sister-in-law of the sperm donor) motioned for us to sit by her and the rest of her family...um, no. As we were deciding where to sit, wouldn't you know it...the sperm donor and the wicked wife walked into the church. They looked right at me right as I was saying I didn't want to sit by certain people for fear of having to sit too close to the sperm donor.

Honestly, I don't think he knew who I was at first. As a matter of fact, most of them didn't know who I was– they thought I was Dennis' girlfriend or date. How pathetic is that? When the ceremony ended, we rushed out the door. As we were standing on the sidewalk waiting to blow the bubbles at the newlyweds, the sperm donor and his wicked wife stood right behind us. It's funny that everywhere I seemed to go that night, he or she was somewhere around me. Talk about being put to the test.

At the reception, Dennis and I sat with my cousin Billy and a guy from high school, Walter. We sat as far away from the sperm donor and the rest of the family as possible. I'm sure they were not happy with Dennis over that one, but I know that he doesn't care. I avoided the entire table at all costs but eventually got sucked in by someone when Dennis and I were standing at the bar, next to their table. I had to use the restroom, so I left my drink with Dennis. When I came out of the bathroom, I saw that Dennis was standing there talking to the sperm donor. I planned to grab my water from the bar and return to my safe haven. Another aunt (sister-in-law of the sperm donor) had been staring at me while I was standing at the bar and finally figured out who I was. Darn. I didn't want to talk to anyone as I didn't have much to say, but I politely stood there and spoke with her for a few minutes. I was kind of offended at first when she started talking to me because she said that she couldn't believe how beautiful I have become...gee, thanks! Anyway, the sperm donor was sitting right next to her, so my eyes were fixated on her, her husband, and Beth the entire time. Not once did I let my eyes connect with his or even move in his direction. Several of them seated at the table were asking me questions about cancer, and I told them about the genetic mutation.

As I started to explain the genetic mutation to my aunt, I could feel the sperm donor was staring at me and hanging on every word that I was saying. As much as I wanted to say, "the genetic mutation came from the person sitting next to you," or "the only thing that the person next to you ever gave me was cancer," I bit my tongue and simply told them that the mutation came from the Ward side. I then offered to send the information from the genetic testing to anyone who wanted it. As my cousin Dennis and I walked away from them, he told me how shocked but proud of me he was for me not saying what I really wanted to say. I had taken the high road and didn't give anyone any reason to speak poorly of me. I think that it would have been easier for me to say what I wanted to say to make it known to the sperm donor that he has shattered my life and that I will forever blame him for all of this. But, I didn't, and that was so hard. Dennis said the sperm donor called him over when I went to the restroom and made a comment about how he is glad to see that I'm doing so well. I thought to myself- he has no idea. He only knows what I want him to see. I wouldn't give him the satisfaction of knowing the pure hell I have been through, how many tears have fallen from my eyes, how I hate what I see when I look in the mirror, how I feel like I will never be good enough for someone to love me, and how I've had hopes and dreams taken away from all because of him. I don't like to say that I'm proud of myself, but in this case, I am. I had the opportunity right in front of me to say what I wanted to say...the door was wide open...but I didn't. What is funny is that never once did he say a single word to me; I think he knew better. I, unfortunately, will see the sperm donor again this summer, as my Aunt Shirley (his sister) is getting married. At least my mom and dad will be at that wedding.

Monday, June 16, 2008
Appointments, Appointments, Appointments

Last week was crazy busy with appointments. I had physical therapy on both Monday and Thursday. My physical therapist wasn't there, so someone else was working with me. She was kind but pushed me beyond my limits and caused me significant pain. I have a few new exercises to increase my range of motion and my strength. She checked my range of motion and seemed pleased with the progress that I'm making, but I'm still weak. I do my PT exercises in my sleep so that probably accounts for some of the progress I have made. I go back Tuesday and Thursday of this week.

On Wednesday, June 11th, I went back to the boobie pumping station for my second fill up. It was pretty uneventful, and I didn't cry again. Wow, having two appointments in a row where I didn't cry is absolutely amazing! When Dr. Gimbel, my plastic surgeon, inserted the needle into the port, I must have made a face because he asked me if I could feel a pinching and I said yes, but not on my chest, in my back. It is so weird that when I touch certain parts of the foobies, I can feel it through my back, but if I touch my back, I can't feel anything. Dr. Gimbel was commenting about how nicely my incisions have healed, and his nurse Judy said, "Beautiful, they are just beautiful." I looked at her with a quizzical expression on my face and said, "Beautiful?? Seriously, now. Come on." She laughed at me and said that beauty is in the eye of the beholder. Yeah, yeah, whatever. My thinking is that they are kind of like parents- they have to say nice things about me. I mean, how horrible would it be of them to say something like, "OMG Melissa, your incisions look terrible. You are all hacked up and just a disaster." Dr. Gimbel seemed to find much humor in me telling him that I wanted to get two new t-shirts made up- one that says Miss Proportioned and another that says Surgical Distortion. I go back on Wednesday for another fill up at the BP station. I seem to be tolerating the fills reasonably well but have been experiencing some muscle spasms and pain with it. I have not gotten to the point of needing the muscle relaxers, yet.

On Thursday, June 12th, I met with my medical oncologist, Dr. Puhalla. She is the new medical oncologist that I started seeing in January. We talked briefly about how things went with the surgery, and she asked me if I was happy with the outcome. Um, not so much. As she was getting ready to examine me, I told her not to be alarmed by what she would see. When she opened my gown, she looked at my incisions on the right side and said, "What is wrong with this? Why don't you like it?" My response was simply, "Because it isn't me. I liked me as I was before all this cancer shit happened."

145

She asked me about my hot flashes and to her amazement and mine, now that I thought about it, I have had only about a handful since I've been off work. My hot flashes were so bad at work sometimes that I would have about one every hour that would last for five minutes or more. I would frequently go out to the secretary in my department, turn her fan on high, and stand there until I was able to get my temperature to drop back down. So yeah, seems as though my hot flashes are stress-induced, and the anti-depressant medication probably wouldn't help with that anyway. I asked Dr. Puhalla when I should start seeing a dermatologist for an annual full-body skin exam since there is a possible link between the BRCA2 mutation and melanoma. She recommended that I start thinking about that now. I think I've put it off because I don't know how I feel about someone seeing every inch of my body...I don't think I have ever seen it all. EEEKKKKK!!!!!!!!!! I will make that appointment sometime in the near distant future. I go back to see Dr. Puhalla in September.

Wednesday, June 18, 2008
Fill-up #3

Today made my third trip to the boobie pumping station. I had to wait for what seemed like an eternity because Dr. Gimbel, my plastic surgeon, was double-booked. My appointment was scheduled for 1:30 pm, but I didn't get into see him until about 2:15 pm. I did my usual routine– go in the room, undress from the waist up, and robe myself with the opening in the front. Then I lay down on the exam table with my feet dangling (which totally drives them crazy) and my iPod in my ears. Dr. Gimbel entered shortly after and made a comment about me being in my standard pose. He left, and Judy entered shortly after to get the sodium chloride ready. She almost kicked my flip-flops right off my feet as to say that it drives her nuts that I leave my feet dangling there. As she was preparing everything, I asked her if she had a tissue expander for me to look at because I was curious to know what was inside of me. After all, I know what the implant looks like. I was very intrigued by the tissue expander. It wasn't much of what I had expected. Some of them are round while others are almost like a kidney shape; I have a round-shaped implant. I sat there and played with it for a few minutes and then gave it back. I thought about asking if I could take it for the week to play with it, but I didn't.

When Dr. Gimbel inserted the needle into the port, I made a comment about how I didn't feel anything this time. I explained that I find it very odd that I could feel it in my back last time, but when I touch my back, I don't feel anything. He said that is because my back is now on my front and I laughed as I told him that I call it my frack. He got a kick out of that one. Then I went into the whole frack thing with him and Judy. They were laughing so hard. As they were cleaning up, Dr. Gimbel said that they were practicing their "routine" as they were thinking about going out on the road and wanted to know if I would join them. I asked if their show was going to be like Krusty the Clown and Side Show Bob (from The Simpsons). He said I could do my frack routine and then I offered to show people the foobies for a fee. I could be their circus freak. I continued to go on about the frack, and then Dr. Gimbel told me of a lady that he had recently seen who was going to have tissue/fat taken from her buttocks. I lost it. I told him I don't think that I would want to tell anyone about that, but to my surprise, he said that people talk about it more than I can imagine. So, I guess she will have a frass. Oh boy, where I could take that! Anyways, that led me to the frick thing. I had left that part out of the frack conversation because I know he already thinks I'm off my rocker. When I explained how one would get a frick and that it would give a whole new meaning to wearing dickies, they were in stitches. It was by far the best appointment I've had there in the year I have been going. Judy kept telling me how funny I am. As I was leaving, she told me to work on getting that other part of the anatomy (frick). I laughed so loud that it echoed through the hallway.

I go back next week for my fourth fill-up, which should be the final one.

Thursday, June 26, 2008
Cancer Crap Update

Happy Graduation to me! I "graduated" from physical therapy last week because I totally kick ass. I have regained most of my range of motion in a mere two and a half weeks, and to think that Dr. Gimbel, my plastic surgeon, gave me eight weeks. Yeah, whatever. I knew that wasn't going to happen. It was a combination of not wanting to do eight weeks of physical therapy and Dr. Gimbel telling me that I needed to work on getting my range of motion back before I started working out again that pushed me to get through the PT as quickly as I could. I still have some work to do but promised I would do my exercises at home to continue to increase my range of motion to get it back to "normal" and I have to start working on some strengthening exercises as I'm still weak in my right arm. Gosh, I can't wait to get back to the gym!

I went to see Dr. Fill Up Me Boobie (aka Dr. Gimbel) again for my fourth boobie pumping. It was the fastest appointment that I've ever had with him. I didn't even have the chance to get "comfortable" in the waiting room before I was taken back. Judy was making fun of me because apparently, I handed the parking lot attendant my appointment card with my money last week. She went to gather up the things needed for my fill, and I went through my usual routine of getting undressed and lying down in my normal position. Dr. Gimbel came in and asked if he could see the foobies. I said, "Maybe!" Then I realized he is the one cutting me with a knife in a few months so I suppose I should comply with his requests. He was a bit concerned with the redness that has developed over the past week. I told him that my scars have been very red lately, but he seemed to think that was okay. It was more the skin above the scar on my right side that concerned him. As he got ready to stab me with the needle, I commented on how I cringe every time he sticks me with the needle, but I don't budge when I get a tattoo, which seems silly to me. Apparently, others have made the same comment to him. He told me companies are now paying to advertise on people's bodies. I told him it was definitely something to consider and he said that I should choose the company wisely if I'm going to tattoo it on my body. I asked him how much he was willing to pay for me to advertise for him. It seems as though the price tag of advertising on my body is beyond what he is willing to pay...his loss.

As he was filling me up, I could feel the pressure and told him how tight the foobie felt. Up to this point, I hadn't felt the pressure and tightness like the last time I went through this. I had a feeling it wasn't going to be a good thing for me. He removed the needle and then repeatedly rubbed the area of my frack that I can feel in my back, which resulted in a combination of laughing and feeling like I might jump out of my skin. It's so weird. This led me to ask him if the girl having the tissue removed from

148

her ass(ets) would feel it in her butt when he touches her foobies. He laughed at me and told me no, but he thought it was hilarious that I sat around for a week wondering about it. I had hoped this would be my last fill, but I have to go back again next week for another one. Dr. Gimbel indicated that over the next year, the muscle will get thinner. Things should smooth out a little bit, but the right side will always be distorted. Blah, blah, blah...yeah, I'm working on dealing with that as soon as I deal with the whole having breast cancer thing.

I went to the grocery store, so I would have something to eat besides yogurt and bananas in my house; though I'm convinced I could live on just that. As I was driving the short seven miles from the doctor's office to the store, I could feel the pain coming on. It is definitely different from the pain that I experienced last year. I'm not having muscle spasms, but the pain is definitely enough to stop me in my tracks. It has gotten worse throughout the evening to the point of my having to take some Tylenol to control the pain. It only took the edge off slightly so I'm not sure what else I can do to get rid of the pain. The Vicodin isn't an option because then I can't drive, and I do need to get around. I tried napping because I'm exhausted, but I couldn't sleep very well because of the pain. I'm sure I will be tossing and turning in pain this evening. It makes me look forward to my appointment next week. Sweetness- more pain and lopsidedness! Life doesn't get any better than that.

Wednesday, July 2, 2008
Back to Work, Back to Life

Well, yesterday was my first day back to work since May 5th. I had been preparing myself for this day by waking up at 5:30 am each morning for the last three weeks, but I was still ten minutes late. My electricity went out on me a few times (even once while I was in the shower, gotta love that). I was excited yet nervous about going back for some reason. For the first time in my life, I didn't worry (too much) about what was going on at work and if they would make it without me (of course they would) while I was on medical leave. It was great to walk in and get such a warm and loving welcome. They truly missed me here. Coming to work gave me a feeling like I have a purpose again. I'd spent the last two months taking care of me, going to endless doctors' appointments, and doing the physical therapy thing. Somehow being at work almost makes me feel somewhat normal. My friend Mike came over to visit and brought me a bag of Reese's Cups, which made my day.

Overall, it wasn't very eventful. I spent a good portion of the day sorting through things, reading my emails, and figure out the new forms that we have to use for special education. I am at work again today, but I have another appointment with Dr. Philip Mebooby at 1:30 pm so depending on how much pain I'm in, I may or may not return. Last week, I was down for about three days with the pain. We shall see what happens. I suspect that we will be setting a date for my next surgery today. I love being at the mercy of my doctors!

Thursday, July 3, 2008
Next BP Station...500 Miles Ahead

Yesterday was my last visit to Dr. Philip Mebooby at the BP Station...at least until my next surgery. It was a long appointment for some reason. I was there for almost two hours. It was rather taxing, but I made the best of the situation and chatted up Dr. Gimbel, my plastic surgeon, and the nurse. Everything was pretty much the standard operating procedure. Lie on the table, find the port, stick me with the needle, and fill 'er up doc. I made a comment twice about the pressure that I was feeling and how tight it was getting. I was half thinking that it was going to implode as he continued to fill it up. That would have been interesting, to say the least. As he was filling me up, the pain began. I said, "Doesn't it make you feel bad that you have to fill me up and cause me pain?" It was a rhetorical question as I had assumed everyone has the same pain that I do, but to my surprise, he said he actually feels awful for me because I am the only one that has ever experienced this amount of pain with the fills, which he attributes to my being "so tiny". I can't win here! He indicated that I need to keep a watchful eye (maybe two) on the radiated skin over the next month to be sure that there are no changes in the appearance or color. This would apparently be bad, very bad. I've had a good bit of pain again, but I am taking Tylenol to try to control it somewhat so that I can at least work. So far, so good.

I had a few questions for him as I've spent some time studying the right foobie. There is a patch of skin inside the football-shaped scar that has hair on it (the rest of it is smooth and hairless from the radiation). For some reason, when I was told he would be taking my latissimus muscle, I didn't necessarily realize that meant that he would be taking the skin that covers it as well. He seemed to find humor in my telling him that the hair bothered me, but then he made me realize that it's a good thing that my back isn't hairy like a guy's back. EEKKK!!!

We scheduled my next surgery to remove the tissue expander and put in the implant for Tuesday, August 19th at Shadyside Hospital. I expressed my concerns with Shadyside, but he assured me that there would be no transporters or mean night nurses involved this time. As he was preparing the paperwork for the next surgery, I asked him what happens after I go for my post-op appointment. Does he not see me again? For as much as I have cried in this man's office and hate all that he has "done" to me, I am worried about not seeing him regularly. I have been in his office more than any other office. He said that he will see me every few months the first year and then annually after that. That is almost comforting.

He then made it a point to remind me that the goal is to make me look as symmetrical as possible in clothing– not naked, not in a bathing suit, but when dressed. I gave him a half-smile and put my head down as I said,

"I know, I know. I'm working on dealing with that." I know that he thinks that I am looking to be perfect. Maybe in a sense that is slightly true, but the reality is that I wish every single day that I could be "ME" again. I wasn't perfect before all of this, but I was me. I guess I figure that since I've had to lose a part of me against my own will in an attempt to save my life, then the least I could have is perfection in the reconstruction. I then asked him the question that I already knew the answer to in hopes of getting a different response.

It still remains that the current surgery guarantees nothing. The implant can shrink again, and I could need another surgery to reconstruct the reconstructed reconstruction. Yeah, that would downright suck. When I asked him if he would take the other latissimus muscle, he said no. I wanted to know the other options, and he said that he would wait for me to gain weight. I laughed at him and said, "Good luck with that. It's not going to happen." I'm sure he knew I was very serious about that.

As much as I wish I would get a month "off" from all this cancer crap, I have my appointment with my gynecological oncologist on July 11th.

Friday, July 4, 2008
Pain, Pain Pills, and Heartache

I made it through most of yesterday at work by popping Tylenol like it was candy. It seemed to take the edge off the pain for a little bit, but by about 2:30 pm, I'd had more than I could handle. It must have been pretty obvious because the secretaries in my department had made a comment to me about not looking well. I came home, took a Vicodin, and passed out for three hours. I was still loopy when I woke up, so I wasn't able to drive to my parent's house as I had intended. I called my Grammy's house to talk to my uncle, but I got my aunt instead. She kept telling me she couldn't understand me because my speech was slurred. I finally told her that I had to take a Vicodin for the pain, so she didn't think I was drunk or doped up on something else.

The pain continued throughout the evening, so I wasn't able to sleep very well. I was hoping that today would be a better day, but the pain is still there, and it's making me miserable. It's like a burning and stabbing kind of pain. I try to massage it in hopes that the pain will stop, but it doesn't, and truthfully, I can't feel anything except for the pain anyways. I'm going to take some Tylenol today because I want to be able to drive to my parents' house to visit with my Uncle Warren and my friend Jenna.

Not only was I in physical pain yesterday, but it was an emotionally exhausting day as well. I had received emails from two of the gals I had met in Las Vegas at the Emerald Dream Ball with news that broke my heart. One has had a recurrence of breast cancer. And the other gal, Crystal, who I had connected with instantly while in Vegas, has a 12mm node on her lung and the doctors think it is that cancer has metastasized. It tore my heart to pieces when I read her email. When I called her, it took everything in me not to break down into tears as I left her a message. She is only a few years older than I am and was diagnosed on April 24, 2007 with Stage IIIA breast cancer. I never wanted to imagine that any of us would have a recurrence or that cancer would metastasize. This serves as a reminder that life truly isn't fair. It is also the exact reason why I tend to be realistic about this whole cancer thing when so many people (especially my mom and dad) refuse to acknowledge that cancer can still be there and could come back with a vengeance. It is the harsh reality of this disease, and not any single one of us has any control over it.

Sunday, July 6, 2008
The SCARProject

I came upon this website today and wanted to be sure others saw it, too. It is emotional and hard to take, even as a breast cancer survivor with similar scars. I know it is hard to understand what someone is going through when you cannot physically see the problem, the damage, or the scars. I think this website will give some insight into what it is that I see every single day when I look in the mirror and why I say that this will never, ever go away.

I would suggest not looking at the site at work, unless it is, behind closed doors with some tissues handy to wipe away the tears. There is a lady that has a football-shaped scar on her right side like I do.

www.davidjayphotography.com/TheSCARProject/

As has been said before, the worst scar that cancer leaves behind is that done to one's self-esteem. This project explains why my self-esteem and self-image has been so traumatized by this disease.

154

Friday, July 11, 2008
Patience and Strength

I don't remember praying for patience today because I know better than that, but today was definitely a test of my patience and strength. I left work at about 2 pm to be at my appointment with my gynecological oncologist, Dr. Kristen Zorn, at 2:30 pm. I got stuck in traffic and had to call the Hillman Cancer Center to let them know I would be late. The lady at the switchboard transferred me to the second floor, Patient Services. As I'm telling the lady that I have an appointment with Dr. Zorn, she repeatedly corrects me on the name. I then tell her over and over that my doctor's last name is Zorn. She argues with me that there is no Dr. Zorn that works at Hillman. I said she is in the high-risk ovarian cancer center. She continues to tell me that Dr. Zorn does not, and she knows this because she has worked at Hillman for twenty-nine years. I'm thinking– what the fuck? I pulled over in my car to grab my cancer resource binder and searched through until I found something with a number. It turned out that Dr. Zorn is on the third floor, not on the second floor. I helped the secretary realize that she does not know everything. She transferred me to the third floor, and all I got was a recording, "Please continue to hold. Your call is important to us." Well, if it is so important, why do I have to continue to hold for five minutes? I never did get in touch with anyone before I got to Hillman. I rushed inside and up to the third floor. I don't like the setup of Hillman because I can't ever remember which pod I'm supposed to go to. A physician was kind enough to help me with that. A nurse came out to talk to me and told me that I did not have an appointment at 2:30 pm. I told her I scheduled it over a month and a half ago. She left and came back a few minutes later to tell me that my appointment was at 9:15 that morning. I told her that I had 2:30 pm written everywhere. She explained that Dr. Zorn and the ultrasound tech had already left for the day so I couldn't get anything done there. Shit! She asked me to wait while she called Magee to see if I could get it done there. As "luck" would have it, Magee was able to get me in today, but they were running about an hour behind schedule. Even though that sucked, I still took it.

The nurse wrote up the script and told me that Dr. Zorn would have the results by Monday. I had a few questions for Dr. Zorn that I wanted to have answered, so I asked that she call me. I explained to the nurse that a physician at a meeting I recently attended indicated that there is no reason for BRCA2 carriers to have their ovaries removed. WHAT??? The nurse seemed disturbed by this and said she would have Dr. Zorn call me to "straighten ME out." It seems like I'm not the one that needs straightening out, but that the doctors need to get on the same page. I had also planned to fight to keep my ovaries because, to be honest, I'm not sure I can handle it.

I sped over to Magee and got there at about 3:30 pm. I had to get registered before I could do anything. Since the lab service was around the corner, I decided I would go there first. The room was filled with pregnant women and new moms. Are you kidding me? I sat patiently for about five minutes before I couldn't take it anymore. I was getting all choked up and wanted to say, "Please stop, I can't emotionally handle listening to anyone talking about having a baby when I have to be reminded that my choice to have a baby was taken from me by fucking cancer!" Yeah...I know...BITTER, table for one!

I left there to go check in at the gynecological center. As I looked around, there were about eight pregnant women with their husbands/boyfriends. Am I being punished today for something?? I signed in there and walked back down to lab services. By that time, most of the women were gone. Anytime I have gone to lab services, the male nurse, Chris, has always been the one to take my blood, so I was not pleased when the female nurse decided she would take me. I knew it was going to be two stabs instead of one. I asked her to use a butterfly, and she told me that she would like to see what I have (veins). I wanted to say, "No, lady, you will use a butterfly!" I kindly asked her that if she doesn't feel like she can use a butterfly that I would like to have Chris come and do it. She seemed offended, but I didn't care. She took her first stab at my left arm. This side has always been problematic for getting blood. I could feel her moving the needle around in my arm, searching for the vein. I knew she wasn't going to get it, but she continued chasing after it. Finally, I think she got the message when I screamed because of the pain. She moved over to the right arm. She had been chatting the whole time and continued to do so. She asked me a ton of questions and only got minimal responses from me. I wanted to say, "Hey toots, pay attention. That's my arm you are shoving a needle into." She was finally able to get the blood for the CA-125 from the right side.

I returned to the gynecological center with two bandages in the crook of both elbows...cute, I know. I sat in the courtyard for almost an hour before I got called back. The nurse was pleasant and made me as comfortable as I could be. As she was preparing my stomach for the ultrasound, she noticed my tattoo (the pink and teal ribbon that make a heart) and made a comment that she liked it. She said it is the only tattoo she has ever seen that she liked. The ultrasound took about seven minutes. I was able to watch everything as the monitor was to my left. There was nothing exciting happening during the ultrasound. Then we did the sonogram. This took about fifteen minutes. I noticed the large black objects on the screen but thought those were my ovaries. In my mind, it was like the mammogram. If there were anything there that shouldn't be there, it would be white. That was not the case, but I didn't realize this until later in the appointment. I watch her mark what I think are my ovaries, and then she started taking sound bites of them. She asked me if I have

156

noticed any difference in my menstrual cycles. I told her that the length of time between them has increased over the past year, and then commented that I can't believe she could tell something was going on. She told me that my endometrial lining is very cystic. That was super exciting since I know that Tamoxifen can cause endometrial cancer. She finished and told me to get dressed, but then changed her mind in case the doctor wanted to take a look. I was coaching myself while she was gone that it would be fine. When she returned with the doctor behind her, I almost lost it. He took another look and said that the black images on the monitor were cysts on my ovaries. OH! I've always had cysts on my ovaries, so I was somewhat relieved until he told me that I needed to have the test repeated in about six to eight weeks. What did I do to deserve this?? I do not like the idea of them shoving that damn probe in my who-ha more than what is absolutely necessary. When all was said and done, I finished up at the hospital at 6 pm. It was definitely an exhausting day that tested my patience and my strength. I seriously feel like I want to crawl up into my bed and stay there for a while with the blankets over my head.

Sunday, July 20, 2008
Happy Birthday to Me!!

Thursday, July 17th was my birthday. Woo Hoo! Happy Birthday to ME! Around this time last year, I was having surgery number three, and I spent my entire birthday lying in bed recovering from surgery from the day before. I had spent the rest of the week being miserable because we had a microburst and my electricity was off for two days, so I was nuclear hot. And Friday of that week, I hit my rock bottom. I had an appointment with Dr. Gimbel and couldn't say anything because I was sobbing. I came home and sobbed the rest of the day and night. I refused to talk to anyone and sat on my back patio rocking back and forth in my chair, crying for hours on end. My friend found me sitting back there and was heartbroken that I had reached such a dark place. So, as I reflected on how I spent my birthday last year, I decided that I was going to celebrate it right this year and make up for last year's missed opportunity.

My birthday celebration started on Wednesday. My friend Annette and I went to Max and Erma's in Shadyside for dinner. She gave me my presents in a purse that looks like a poodle and it may be the most ridiculous thing I have ever seen, (I had given it to her for her birthday!) She got me a little ducky flashlight for my keychain...not to use in the dark but to light up my implants. Oh yeah, it is something to see...they glow! HA! She had a t-shirt made up that says MISS PROPORTIONED! After dinner and dessert, we did some shopping.

On Thursday, I went into work for a half-day. My friend Naomi called me out into the hallway, and I was surprised to see most of the people in the office standing there. They sang happy birthday to me, which always embarrasses me. The ladies in my department got me a Victoria's Secret gift card, and we all had some healthy treats. Before I left work, I, unfortunately, had to go to a funeral for a youngster that I worked with two years ago when she entered kindergarten. After the funeral, I went to South Hills Village to meet my cousin Dina for lunch. We went to Roxy's, which was pretty good and then we did some shopping. I got a ton of birthday wishes via email, MySpace, text messages, and phone calls. It was GREAT!

On Friday, I had planned a "Cancer Can Kiss My Ass Happy Hour and Birthday Bash" at the Pleasure Bar in Bloomfield. I had invited some people and was interested to see who would show up. I wasn't sure what was going to happen when my worlds collided, but it was a great time. My cancer cronies, Noella, Jay, and Jerry, came, along with Noella's friend Craig and Jay's friend, Chong. Jenna, my friend from high school, and her husband were there. My friend Mike from Edinboro showed up. My friend Christina from work and her friend, Francesca, were also there and my cousin Dennis came a little later. I was happy to see that everyone seemed to get along well, and we talked about everything under the sun!

I decided that I would do one shot but ended up having a Red Death and a shot. It took me almost two hours to drink the Red Death. I could definitely feel it since I haven't had a drink for well over a year. I figured one drink wouldn't kill me, at least it better not! By around 10:00 pm, the only people left were me, Jay, Chong, and Mike. I decided that I would go with Jay and Chong to the Cabana Bar in Cranberry. It was totally crazy. I initially wore my tiara, but after being asked for the fifth time if I was getting married, I decided to take it off. I ended up staying until almost 1 and didn't get home and into bed until 1:30 am. Whew! It has been a long time since I have done that. I used to be a pro at that, but I'm so out of the game now.

On Saturday I went to see the family and I had a graduation party to go to. I stopped to see my mom, and we decided to go to the farmer's market. I didn't get to see my dad because he was out golfing. The nerve! I went to see my Aunt Aggie before I went to the graduation party. I had planned to be at the party by 4:00 pm but I fell asleep on my Aunt's couch for almost two hours. I was so beat from the night before. I got to the graduation party at about 5:30 pm or so. I pretty much hung out with my friend Jenna. At this point, her family probably thinks that I'm somehow related because I'm always around for family events. She gave me a Mattress Factory (art museum) t-shirt, which totally excited me because I so want to be an MFer!!! Her mom gave me the Steelers blanket that she finished making for me because I was "whining" that it wasn't done.

On Sunday, my best friend, Ken, stopped over to see me. I haven't seen him for two weeks, so it was nice to hang out for a little bit with him. I went to church, and then I treated myself to a piece of the Oakmonter (from the Oakmont bakery...it is half chocolate cake and half cheesecake and is amazing!) as my birthday present to myself. I am going out to dinner with my friend Gina on Tuesday to celebrate my birthday with her.

I had a wonderful birthday (week) with my family and friends. I think I definitely made up for my crappy birthday last year!

Wednesday, July 30, 2008
Pre-operative Appointment

Today at 11:15 am, I went for my pre-operative appointment with my primary care physician. As I prepared for this morning, I decided I would be proactive and drink a ton of water (seven glasses to be exact) before I went so that there would be no trouble stabbing my little veins for some blood. Wishful thinking, I know.

The appointment was pretty much like all of the other pre-operative appointments. I couldn't wait to be called back to pee in the cup. I think my teeth were floating. The receptionist kindly got me into a bathroom and gave me a cup. It was full to the brim and beyond. I was called back a few minutes later. I was happy about that because a lady was sleeping in the waiting room and she was snoring so loud. As luck would have it...I forgot my iPod today.

I went with the nurse. She checked my blood pressure, heart rate, weight, and height. She gave me a gown and asked me to change from the waist up and then left the room. Before I could do anything, she was back to check my temperature. As I was opening the gown, she pulled it away from me and said, "Here let me help you with that. It goes like this." I looked at her with my "WTF??" look on my face. As much as I wanted to remind her that I have been to many doctor visits and have never needed her assistance or anyone else's assistance in figuring out how to put the gown on, I impatiently waited for her to leave the room so that I could change.

I changed and waited only a few minutes for Dr. Andrews, my PCP, to come in for the rest of the exam. He did his regular routine– asked what medication I'm on, asked if I'm having any problems, asked if I'm allergic to anything, blah, blah, blah. He knows the answers to every single one of those questions. Stop asking me and read my chart! As he was checking my lungs, I think he noticed my scar on my back and pulled my gown back further so that he could check it out. I wanted to say, "Hey, if you think that is something to see, you should check out the other eight scars. They are really pretty." But I refrained.

I asked Dr. Andrews about the need for blood work. He thought I needed it but wasn't sure because he couldn't read Dr. Gimbel's handwriting. He could decipher that a urinalysis and a pregnancy test were needed, but the pregnancy test is to be done the day of surgery. I laughed and said that Dr. Gimbel should know better. It is not humanly possible for me to be pregnant...that would require a man and well, um, no one has replied to my newspaper ad (maybe because I never actually posted it, but that is beside the point).

160

Dr. Andrews gave me the name of a dermatologist so I can go do the whole skin cancer check crap. Woo Hoo. As he left the office, he said, "No offense, but I don't want to see you for a while." Hey buddy, trust me. The feeling is mutual with you and all of my doctors.

I had to wait for the nurse to come back in to take my blood. I had hoped that it would be a one-shot deal, but it never works the way I want it to. She checked both arms twice and wasn't seeing anything. I started slapping my arms, trying to wake up my veins, but that didn't do much of anything. I told her that if she thought she couldn't get it, she shouldn't bother; I would go to Magee to have it done because I don't want her chasing my veins. The nurse thought she could get it from my right arm and promised that if she couldn't get it, she would pull it out. I let her try...no luck. She said that she would get someone else to try if I was okay with it.

I was moved to the room where they draw blood and had to wait for the other nurse. She checked both arms and wasn't seeing much either. She asked me if I had any water this morning and seemed shocked when I told her that I'd already had seven glasses of water (and that doesn't include what I had at home when I was working out). I suggested a heated compress, but I got the impression that she didn't like me telling her what to do. She refused to use a butterfly needle on me because in her words, she "would be there all day." Funny, I'm not there all day when anyone else uses a butterfly. I decided to suck it up and try it so that I didn't have to drive to Magee. The only thing I can say about anyone else ever trying to stick a regular-sized needle in my arm is TO HELL WITH THAT!!! I could feel everything she did with it, and I seriously thought I was going to cry or pass out. Yeah, call me a baby. Whatever, I'm cool with it. She was finally able to get it after some pushing in, pulling out bullshit. She told me that I could curse at her, and though I really did want to because I told her to use the butterfly, I didn't. I won't ever let her come near me with a needle again.

Not that I'm actually counting but twenty more days until surgery number five. Boy, this shit is starting to get REAL old, REAL fast. Oh, wait. It was old a long time ago.

I have officially made it through 372 days of my Tamoxifen. Only 1453 days to go!

Sunday, August 10, 2008
Cancer Sucks

Yesterday morning I woke up hating cancer and the world. It was one of those days that I should have spared the human race and locked myself in my apartment, but I had a lot going on, so I couldn't. I refused to get out of bed when I woke up since I still had an hour before the alarm would go off, so I turned on the television. Bad idea. To magnify my pissed off mood by about ten, I stopped on the St. Jude infomercial and laid in my bed crying for those little babies that have been affected by this disease and also partly for myself. It is a harsh disease, no matter the age. Young or old, it still sucks!

I had about a million thoughts running through my head and wanted it all to stop, but it wouldn't. It never does. Lately, I've been experiencing significant body image issues related to the scarring. Just when I think I might be okay with being in a relationship with someone, I remember that I have a ton of scars all over my upper body and can't imagine why anyone in this world would choose me over someone normal. I'm not naïve enough to believe that sexual and physical attraction is not a large part of an intimate relationship. I know better. My friends and family are sweet for trying to convince me otherwise.

My thoughts were also consumed by the idea that in about twenty-two months, I will be expected to make the decision to have my ovaries removed. I became angry as I thought about my never having children and the fact that there is one girl in particular who doesn't take care of her two kids. She had the oldest one taken away from her, and the newborn baby is so tiny because of her drug usage that he has to wear baby doll diapers. I can't conceptualize why things like this happen. Not that I think I would be the perfect mother, but I'd like to think that I would take better care of my babies.

I finally got out of bed at about 9:00 am, ate something, and then went to the gym in hopes of working out some of my bitchiness. That didn't work. I went about my day trying hard not to say or do anything to offend anyone. Trust me, it was hard. I met my friends for lunch and then headed toward Burgettstown for my aunt's wedding. I stopped at my mom and dad's place before the wedding and was miserable. Sometimes I think my family and friends don't understand that I have bad days because of all of this. Yeah, I put up this great front that I'm okay ninety-nine percent of the time; I act like everything in the world is as it should be, but the reality is that my world is not as it should be and sometimes, I come crashing down. I half thought about going home and crawling back into bed. It's safer for me, and the world, if I'm there on days like this.

I sucked it up and went to the wedding. I was somewhat nervous about it because the sperm donor was there. I had texted my cousin and told him that I was in a bitchy mood and that he might want to forewarn the sperm donor to maintain a safe distance from me. We were seated about two tables back from his, which was too close for comfort, in my opinion. I was agitated because of that, and then I noticed the ashtrays on the tables. Great...so I am already pissed off, I have to worry about if the sperm donor is going to talk to me, and I also have to inhale everyone's cigarette smoke. My bed was sounding better by the second.

I didn't talk to anyone outside of those I speak to on a regular and consistent basis, which might have been about ten people. I spent most of my time talking with my cousin Dennis, who, by the way, everyone thinks is my husband (WTF??). There were several people from the FF's side of the family there that I hadn't seen in years, though I didn't talk to any of them. I'm not sure how I can explain this, but I think an analogy might work. When I was younger, all of these people were a part of my life, kind of. As I got older, I started to drift away from that side of the family and hadn't been around them since I was in high school. They don't know anything about me other than I'm the young breast cancer girl and I don't know much about them either. Being there with them was kind of like having an old pair of jeans that I used to fit into but don't anymore. No matter how hard I try to make the jeans fit, they don't. They are too tight and uncomfortable. I'm sure everyone thought I was a stuck-up bitch but, in my head, if we haven't talked in that long, why now? Because I have cancer? Spare me the sympathy. I don't want it.

There were two occasions when I came into close contact with the sperm donor. As I was walking by the bar, he was standing there but initially had his back to me. I thought I was safe, but then he noticed me and turned in my direction. I looked past him and walked right by him. He kind of had this look of anticipation as though I might stop and talk to him. Did he think I was going to stop and say something to him? Not so much. I went to get a picture with my aunt, and as soon as the sperm donor noticed that I was sitting up there with her, he came over to the table. It took everything in me not to get up and walk away though I really, really wanted to. I was hoping that he wouldn't say anything to me because I'm not sure that I would have been able to control my tongue this time. All of my anger, hurt, frustration, and pain from all this cancer shit goes back to him...the one person in this world that I have the least amount of tolerance for. It is his fault that this happened to me, and as if I didn't have enough harsh feelings toward him before, it is even worse now. Thankfully, he simply asked a stupid question of my aunt and walked away. Hopefully, this will be one of the last encounters I have with him, ever.

As I started thinking to myself, while watching some of the other people there that are battling or have battled cancer get drunk to the point of not being able to stand up straight and inhaling cigarettes like it's nobody's business, I decided it was time to leave. It was hard for me to stand there and watch this kind of behavior without saying something. I understand that everyone deals with things in their own way but using the cancer card for stupid behavior (like drinking instead of taking your cancer meds or your antibiotics) is not acceptable. The fact that we all have the genetic mutation for cancer is all the more reason to avoid those things, so before I offended anyone, I left.

The drive home was not an easy one. I wanted so badly to cry (sob actually), and I'm not even sure why. Well, I do, but it's been the same reason for the last year and a half. I wondered when this will get easier. Will it ever get easier? I wanted to go home and have Justin standing at my door, waiting for me with his arms wide open to take me in and shut the world out for a little while. I wanted him to be there to protect me from it all but, as usual, I came home to nothing, crawled in bed, and continued to wish that, for once, I didn't have to do this on my own.

Tuesday, August 12, 2008
Tightness in My Foobie

I called my plastic surgeon's office because I have been noticing that I'm getting tight on the right side again. It's been about a week or so that I started feeling the pressure, but it was very apparent to me last night as I was running on the treadmill. I can feel the tightness in my chest and in my back, much more than last time, especially now that I'm missing my whole latissimus muscle. It feels like at any given point in time, the incision sites might rip right open again. I'm also losing my range of motion in my right arm again even though I have continued my exercises since being discharged from physical therapy. Judy, the nurse, thought it would be a good idea for me to go in to see Dr. Gimbel tomorrow to be on the safe side and make sure that we are still "all systems go" for the surgery next Tuesday. I have an appointment at 3:30 pm.

As of right now- it is T-minus six and a half days until surgery number five.

Thursday, August 14, 2008
All Systems Go

I went to see Dr. Gimbel, my plastic surgeon, yesterday to have him take a look at the right side to be sure that we are good to go for the surgery on Tuesday. I'd be really ticked off if I had gone to the hospital on Tuesday only to have him say that we couldn't move forward with the surgery. He indicated that there is definitely some tightness (trust me, I know) but it does not visually appear to be shrinking, which I would agree with. I only feel like it is shrinking again because of the pressure I feel in my frack and back, which recently started. He feels the tightness has a lot to do with the fact that I have such thin skin (this would be confirmed by the fact that I can see the blue dye on the inside of the tissue expander through my skin...yeah creepy).

He recommended that we go forward with the surgery on Tuesday and let things take its course. Should the tissue continue to shrink and cause the implant to harden again, we will need to do some "revisions." In his head, he feels that I would have to undergo another surgery on both sides to reduce the size of the implants. In my head, other alternatives need to be considered. The larger the implants, the more tightness I'm likely to experience though I could still experience tightness with smaller implants as well. He knows where I stand on having a smaller implant thing– not going to happen. Being the same size I was before all of this surgery has boosted my self-esteem (only slightly, but it's still a boost) and I'm not about to go backward! In addition to that, the left side would have extra skin that would crinkle if the implants were reduced and that would not sit well with me. I have been a good little patient up to this point and have done all of what has been recommended to me by my doctors. Well, the defiant side of me that has always been there (the side that lives life and does things on my own terms) is starting to take over. I will stand for nothing short of what I want, and smaller implants are not what I want. I almost burst into tears as we talked about the smaller implants but was able to hold it in because I'm so tired of crying over this stuff. I told Dr. Gimbel that all of this cancer shit is wearing me thin, and he said "literally." I wanted to say, "Hey buddy, I make the jokes around here...not you," but I smiled and agreed. It was funny, but not at the time.

I will go forward with the surgery at this point and see what happens to the right side. I'm hoping that since Dr. Gimbel pumped me up slightly more than what is actually needed to allow for some "wiggle room," when the implant is put in, all will be fine. I have decided to stop doing any type of exercise that might use my chest or back muscles for the next four to six months (or until I have a training camp for the Pink Steel Dragon Boating team in April). I haven't been doing the chest flies or the bench press as he recommended, but there are some exercises that I do that indirectly target those areas. I hate to cut back on my workouts because I am starting to see that my body is getting back into shape and it feels/looks good.

I decided yesterday that I am moving. I am going to the next town over to the east. I wanted a bigger, cheaper place, so I got a duplex in Blawnox. It has a garage, full basement, laundry room, two bedrooms, living room, one bathroom, a full kitchen, and an office area (in Melissa's world, this equates to an exercise room). I have decided to go back to school. I start classes on August 26th at the University of Pittsburgh to work toward a master's degree in Social Work. I'm looking forward to it but am a bit nervous that I will be back in school with all of the other things I have going on in my life.

Monday, August 18, 2008
T-minus 10 Hours to Surgery

Well, here it is...surgery number five is upon me in approximately ten hours. I have to be at the hospital at 5:15 am (I'm not sure why they enjoy torturing me), and surgery is at 7:30 am. I'm not sure how long it will take, but I imagine I will be home by early afternoon, as long as all goes well. The pre-op nurse called me today at work, but I missed her call. When she returned my phone call, she asked for Marcia Ward. That made me nervous, but she said that she couldn't hear the message (I would imagine my chart would have been right there or maybe my name was on a list of people to call that day, I don't know). She asked me all the standard questions...if I'm allergic to anything, to which I responded, "Yes, beer, but I don't imagine I can get any of that tomorrow, huh?" Then she said, "Drugs?" and I said, "Recreational." She at least found the humor in that. She gave me the standard speech...no eating or drinking after midnight (so I'm currently eating Reese's Cups because I always figure if I die, at least I had something I enjoyed before I went...yeah, morbid I know), shower with anti-bacterial soap in the morning, no fingernail polish, and no makeup. When she said no makeup, I said "yeah, yeah, yeah" knowing full well in my head that I will be there with it on tomorrow.

The plan is for my parents, aunt, and Grammy to meet me at the hospital at 5:15 am. I have this thing with needing to be alone the night before surgery, though right now I do kind of wish that Justin was here. Why does stupid Las Vegas have to be so far away? My dad is planning to spend the night with me tomorrow and actually said he would be staying until Friday or Saturday. I attempted to convince him that he only needed to stay for one night but then finally had to tell him the truth is I can't handle his snoring for that many days in a row, so he has to go home on Wednesday. I will be fine, and if I need something, Annette is close by and will be here for me.

I realized that this surgery has actually crept up on me much faster than I had anticipated. I feel like it was yesterday that I had the last operation, and now here we are again. I know this surgery isn't a big deal, but I'm actually dreading it more than any of the previous surgeries. I think a lot of it has to do with the fact that I'm tired of it all. My hope, strength, and will are starting to waver. I'm trying hard to keep going strong, but I'm so exhausted and drained from all of this. My heart is so heavy with hurt and anger, my emotions are on high, and physically, I'm done with having my body mutilated. It's been almost one year and five months to the day since this all started, and I feel like I haven't been able to catch my breath since that time. When things almost feel like I'm getting back on the right track, I start readjusting to my new normal, and I begin working on trying to come to terms with my physical appearance, something comes up again, and I'm back at square one. It's like the cancer is its own little being within me that every so often keeps rearing its ugly little head to remind me of how damned annoying it is and how much control over my life it has.

Wednesday, August 20, 2008
Surgery #5

Yesterday, August 19th, I got up at 4:00 am to get ready for my surgery. I took my anti-bacterial soap shower and removed my toenail polish. Despite being told not to, I put some makeup on. I was nervous, so I was texting Justin to create a distraction for myself. Luckily, he is a night owl and was able to entertain me. I left the house by 4:40 am and planned to be at the hospital early, but as soon as I crossed the Highland Park bridge, I realized I forgot my prayer shawl. I have never gone into surgery without it. I had to turn around to go get it. Thankfully, there isn't a whole lot of traffic this time of the morning. I made it back home by 4:50 am and was gone again in less than a minute. I made it to the hospital at about 5:10 am and was immediately checked in and taken up to pre-op. My parents, aunt, and Grammy were already there. I didn't even get a chance to say hi to my aunt and Grammy before I was swept away.

I spent about an hour lying on the gurney in the pre-op room before anyone came in to see me. I wanted my family there with me. Usually, I text message my best friend during this time, but I wasn't able to do that, so I was pretty much beside myself. The nurse came in to attempt the IV. She looked at both hands and knew right away that I was going to be a challenge. She asked if I had any secrets for her, and I told her to get a heated compress. It helped a little bit, but she wasn't confident that she would get it, so she didn't even try (I liked her). She decided that the IV team should be called. I repeatedly asked when my family could come to be with me. Finally, they were brought up at about 6:45 am. As soon as they got there, Dr. Gimbel arrived. He asked me if I was ready, I told him that I was not. He asked if I was somewhat prepared, I again said I was not. Dr. Gimble asked if I wanted to go home. My response was, "Yes, bye." He asked my family to leave the room so that he could put a "Y" on my right side. When I said, "Why?", he giggled. I think he was trying to get me to relax a little bit by asking me what types of songs I was listening to. I told him that I always listen to my cancer comfort songs, which are totally depressing but tap into my raw emotions. He said he would see me in a little bit, and I told him he would unless the IV team didn't show (I was totally crossing my fingers that they wouldn't). A short time later, someone from anesthesia showed up. As she was preparing for my IV, I started to cry and asked my dad to come over so that I could hold his hand. She numbed my hand, which hurt just as much and then she put the IV in. I think I was squeezing my dad's hand too hard because he forced me to loosen up my grip. Shortly after, I was given something through the IV to help me relax, and after getting kisses from the family, I was taken off into surgery. The lady from anesthesia tried to convince me to leave my prayer shawl, but I refused. She said it might get iodine on it or it may not come back at all. I told her that I absolutely had to have it with me, and she didn't argue with me anymore about it.

169

As I was being transported to the surgical room, I felt like they were taking me to the back loading dock or something. It didn't look much like a room where surgery would be performed but apparently, it is. I moved from the gurney to the surgical table and was knocked out fairly quickly after that. The operation only took approximately an hour (according to my family), but I was in recovery for a very long time. I remember coming in and out of it many times during the four hours that I was in recovery. I remember the gurney being so darn uncomfortable that I couldn't lie on my back. I was able to roll myself over onto my left side and stayed there for quite some time. I was having a lot of pain on the right side because Dr. Gimbel used the top incision line where I actually have some feeling, and for some reason, my arm hurt like hell too. I think I asked for pain medication about five times. At one point, I heard the nurse say that I was ready to be taken to the step-down recovery room, but then I never went. She told me that my blood pressure had dropped significantly (60 over 40 something). It didn't register until later when I recalled a physician in high school telling me that my blood pressure was so low, he was shocked I was still alive (and it was a good bit higher than 60 over 40 something). Good thing I was too out of it at that point, otherwise I might have panicked. The nurse pushed fluids through my IV for almost two hours before my blood pressure went back up. I wasn't able to get any pain meds while I was being pushed with fluids, which sucked.

At approximately 12:30 pm, I was taken to the step-down recovery room. By that time, I had to pee so bad that I was ready to burst. The nurse offered me a bedpan while in the recovery room, but I just have a bad mental image of that whole situation, so I decided to hold it until I could use a regular bathroom. My parents were brought up after approximately ten minutes. I had gotten some ginger ale because my stomach was feeling a bit weak and then later asked for some crackers. I also asked for some additional pain medication. You know it had to hurt because last time they had to pretty much shove it down my throat. I couldn't lie on the gurney anymore, so I decided it was time to get up. Despite being somewhat nauseous, I wanted to go home and rest on my chaise lounge. I was only in step-down for approximately one hour before I was ready to go. We got back to my apartment at 2:00 pm and crashed. It felt so good to be comfortably resting on my own furniture. I was in and out of awareness for most of the evening. I took two Vicodin throughout the night. My dad stayed over to be sure that I would be okay.

Today, my dad helped me to get some more of my things packed up for the move at the end of the month. I did what I could, but that wasn't a whole lot. I am in much more pain than what I anticipated, but I refuse to take any more Vicodin because that means I can't drive. I'm not able to shower until tomorrow, and I can't wash my hair (wow, does that totally suck). I was given specific instructions of no strenuous exercise until after I see Dr. Gimbel (boy, does he know me well, or what?). I'm going to attempt to take a bath and wash my hair...It should be interesting.

Thursday, August 21, 2008
Removing the Dressing

Today was the day that I was instructed to remove the dressing and shower. I had put it off for most of the evening but finally around 10:00 pm, I decided that I should get it over with. There was a part of me that thought about how I had responded to the unveiling in July 2007, and I didn't want to have to deal with that all over again. It was the day that I entered into a terrifying and dark place with myself. At least I had a better idea of what to expect this time and felt as though I was somewhat more prepared, but I honestly don't think that I'm ever as "prepared" as I'd like to think I am.

I decided the easiest way to remove the dressings would be to get in the shower and pull the tape off from the most sensitive areas to the least sensitive areas as quickly and painlessly (yeah, right) as possible. I have to wonder if I'm slightly sensitive to the tape they use because I have little red bumps where the tape was, and it's very itchy. The incision didn't look all that bad, though I really can't tell because there is steri-strip covering it and I'm not sure if I'm to remove that as well. I would prefer Dr. Gimbel remove it because the sound of tearing it off makes me nauseous.

I stood in the shower staring down at my "new and improved" right foobie. (I think I have discovered the only thing in this world that can actually be considered "new and improved"). I'm not sure why it looks and feels so different from the left side, but it does. It's like a foreign foobie. As much as I had hoped that I wouldn't be overly emotional about all of this, but that was not the case. The reality of all that I have been through hit me square in the face (as if it hadn't a thousand times before). I stood there in awe, wondering how my life ever became such a mess and why I was being robbed of so many precious and private things. It was almost like an out-of-body experience...really. Like I was looking at this body that I was not familiar with, even though it's what I have been dealing with for more than a year now. Somehow, I still can't believe that this is all really, truly happening to me. I could feel myself becoming angry and hurt all over again but not only for me this time. As I continued to stand there looking at myself, I started thinking about Justin, as well. He has never seen the foobies, and I have my doubts that he ever will, but I began to become angry at myself that I could be so selfish to consider allowing him to be a part of this. He doesn't deserve to have someone that has been completely mutilated. I know how angry he would be with me right now if he actually read this, but I can't stop myself from feeling like it's not fair to him because it's not. It's not fair to me, but I can't control that. It's also not fair to him and that, I can prevent.

I got out of the shower and as I was drying off, noticed that I had tape on my shoulders as well. I'm not sure what they were doing to me, but I'm going to have to inquire about that one. I stood in the mirror looking at myself, which is a rare occasion within itself. I tried to touch the right foobie, but it is still a little sensitive. As I was taking note of the difference in the look, feel, size, and shape between the two sides, I longed for nothing more than to be me again. I would give anything in this world if only I could have back what was rightfully mine. Though I'm hardly in the place I was last year with all of this, I'm still having a hard time accepting that this is my reality. THIS is MY body.

Friday, August 29, 2008
Post-op Appointment

I had my post-op appointment with Dr. Gimbel, my plastic surgeon, on Wednesday at 10:00 am. It was a relatively easy and painless appointment, probably one of the fastest I have ever had. He indicated that the right side is healing well, and he confirmed that I must have had a reaction to something because I still have the little red bumps, which he suspects will go away soon. As he approached me to remove the steri-strip, I plugged my ears. He stepped back as if I were entirely off the wall and asked, "What is that about?" I told him I don't like the sound of the steri-strips being pulled off and he giggled at me. He continued to laugh about this after he took it off and threw it away. In his expert, male, plastic surgeon opinion, he is happy with the outcome of the surgery and indicated that I have good symmetry. He didn't even ask what I thought...probably because he gets the same response every time: I want me back. I asked him about the difference in the feel between the two sides, and he confirmed my idea that it is because the skin on the right side is thinner. I seriously feel like at any given point in time, my implant might fall out onto the floor. I'm afraid that if someone hugs me too hard, the implant might go flying out.

He wants to see me in ten weeks. I would be okay with this except he was very stern with me in that I'm not allowed to run or do any high impact exercise until I see him again. UGH! In two weeks, I'm permitted to do "mild bouncy" activities, but I have to wear two sport bras to keep those puppies strapped in. (This, by the way, only further supports my silly idea that it might fall out. It won't fall out, but I could end up lopsided. I'm not sure which is worse, really.) I tried hard to catch him off guard and say that I could run in two weeks, but he is too quick. I am permitted to do strength training and ride the bike...not my idea of a great workout but I guess I will take what I can get right now.

I asked about my identification card for the left implant, as I had recently received the one for the right implant in the mail. Yes, the implants come with their own identification cards and their own serial numbers (which is how I will be referring to them from now on). I'm not sure what I would ever actually use this for, though it says to use it in an emergency. I have no idea what kind of emergency would warrant me flashing my implant identification cards. Somehow, I think if I'm in an emergency situation, the last thing I might be thinking about is whipping them out (the cards, not the implants...though probably those, too). But, hey, whatever. His office has to contact Shadyside Hospital to obtain that card, as it should have been provided to me in May. Before he left to go enjoy some of the zucchini bread I brought, I told him he thoroughly disrupts my workout routine, and I don't appreciate it. He didn't seem to care much.

My next appointment with him is on November 5th. The secretary could hardly believe that she would not be seeing me until that time. They have become accustomed to seeing me there almost weekly since April 2007. I have shed more tears in their office than anywhere else, and they have given me more hugs than most people, so it does kind of feel like I'm leaving my family temporarily. But truth be known, I'm tired of seeing doctors for all this cancer crap, so it is kind of refreshing for me at the same time.

I have come up with two new ideas for t-shirts. I think I need to get a business going here. The first is "I'm the most fun you can have with a flashlight." This is great only if you know that the implants light up if a flashlight is placed under them. Yeah, go ahead and try it; I'm not lying. The second one is, "My scars are better than Evel Knievel's."

Sunday, September 14, 2008
An Overdue Update

I haven't had a whole lot going on medically other than not being able to work out and still feeling like the right implant might fall out. I've started wearing two sports bras to put these puppies on lockdown. I have an appointment with my medical oncologist at the beginning of October for a routine check-up and then the radiation oncologist and my plastic surgeon at the beginning of November. I'm still having some pain in my back, but outside of that, I'm pretty good.

Life has been pretty crazy as of late, and for once, it has nothing to do with cancer or surgeries. I started school at Pitt at the end of August. I am taking two classes and enjoy them. I do have a lot of reading to do for one class, but overall, I think I got pretty lucky with my professors. I don't have any tests in one of my classes and only a mid-term and final exam in the other.

I moved into my new place at the start of this month. For being so excited about moving, I was a mess that day. I have never been one to deal with change very well, and any disruption in my life causes significant stress for me. I was sick to my stomach all day, and I think my mom was afraid that I might have a nervous breakdown. I have some odd nervous habits that I don't realize I display, and it had her a little freaked out, I think. I'm pretty much settled in, though I still have some boxes to go through and I don't know when I will have the time to do that.

Despite everything that I'm worried about, (mainly, being in a large place and living alone with higher bills) I'm actually comfortable here. There is something about this place that reminds me of the house I owned in Edinboro, and I loved that house. For the first time in three years, I'm actually sleeping through the night. I am dreaming again, and I don't hear the 3:00 am train go through, even though I'm almost literally right on top of the railroad tracks. It has been refreshing for me.

Through all of this, I realized something much more profound about myself- I'm ready to figure out where I'm meant to be and to settle in for a while, with someone. Recently, someone told me that I bounce around so much that it is virtually impossible for anyone to get to know me, and I realize that person is right. Once I start feeling comfortable with someone, I disrupt my whole life and change everything (funny for someone that doesn't deal well with change). I've always been afraid of letting myself get comfortable with someone and settling in for the duration. But I realize something is missing in my life– someone to share it with.

I wrecked my car the first week that I moved into my new place. This might be upsetting to most people, but right after I did it, I laughed. I laughed the whole way to work, all the way to the car dealership, the entire time I was in the collision center, and all the way back to the office. I did about eighteen hundred dollars worth of damage, but it was stupid. I couldn't do anything but laugh. I think that this day made me realize how much my perspective on life has truly changed. Pre-breast cancer Melissa would not have dealt well with this. I remember sobbing because of a flat tire on my six-year-old car, and now here I am laughing my ass off that I drove my fairly new car into the garage. Though I have been told that it is okay to have normal responses to crappy things, I can't do that when I look at the grand scheme of things. It is a car, and it can be fixed. This was a walk in the park in comparison to the whole cancer thing.

Last Tuesday I did a video shoot with Clear Channel Communications for the Haute Pink Party on October 4, 2008. It is an event sponsored by UPMC, and it benefits the Susan G. Komen Foundation this year. The ladies at Susan G. Komen gave them my name and said I would be a good person to interview because I have a compelling story to tell. I was surprised because after seeing the Ford Warrior video, I'm shocked anyone would ever want me to speak on camera again; I was a mess!!

Thursday, October 2, 2008
"Feel Your Boobies and Save the Ta-Tas" Month

I had an appointment with my medical oncologist, Dr. Puhalla, today for my routine three-month "feel up." How appropriate during breast cancer awareness month. It was pretty much the run-of-the-mill appointment though I got felt up twice today, by two different people. Though one might think that it would be "exciting" to get felt up twice in one day, the level of discomfort I have when someone touches the foreign objects (especially with any degree of pressure) makes me cringe and want to jump right out of my skin. It results in me holding my breath and making funny faces (oh, boy! How special will that be for Mr. "I'm so lucky even to be close to the foobies" when he decides he should touch them...EEK!).

As far as they can tell from merely copping a feel, things seem to be okay. Dr. Puhalla sat and talked with me at great length about what had been going on since my last visit to her. Since I had been through my annual ovarian cancer screening, I had to bring that up even though it is my least favorite topic. She seemed to question why it is that I am only being screened once a year instead of every six months considering the genetic mutation (Funny thing...I wondered the exact same thing, but I must admit that if I can get away with them shoving that damn probe with the cold gel on it into the who-ha once a year, I'm not going to complain too much about it). She seemed to think that it might be because of my young age and thought maybe the screening would be done every six months after I turn 35 until I told her that I seem to be getting pressured into having my ovaries removed by then. This started the conversation that I'd rather not have. Seriously, I think I would rather chew on glass or bang my head off a wall repeatedly than to have the "baby" conversation one more time.

Since she is my new medical oncologist, and I really, really do like her, I had the conversation. She wanted to know what my thoughts were on having kids, so I told her that I'm working on letting go of that thought because I think it is morally wrong to have children knowing that I'm a BRCA2 carrier (this is my own personal belief, and I have no ill feelings toward those that do have kids). She asked me about harvesting eggs and the genetic testing of the egg before being inseminated. Yep, thought about that too. I have a problem with understanding why I would take Tamoxifen to suppress the estrogen in my body to then have a fertility specialist highjack my body with estrogen to produce eggs. I see that as a considerable risk for a recurrence that I'm not willing to take. I don't want to run the risk of feeding those evil bastard cancer cells– so no pregnancy and no harvesting eggs for me. This brought up the question of why I'm so hell-bent on not giving up my ovaries and fallopian tubes and whatever else they might decide to dig out of my who-ha. Honestly, I'm not ready. It's been a hard year and a half for me, and I'm still dealing day in and day out with the whole breast cancer issue. Let's add to that, more missing parts of what makes me female, pre-mature menopause, weight gain, and a host of other things on top of all the breast cancer stuff. I imagine that is the cocktail for an extremely emotionally/psychologically unstable Melissa. No thanks. My other reason I gave her was that "I'm a self-centered little bitch." Yep, I am; but, I'm okay with it. I'm not ready to deal with the side effects that will come along with having this surgery so as of right now, I'm NOT doing it. She seemed to think that was reasonable...finally someone NOT pressuring me to do this. I was so relieved. While I was meeting with the doc, the other person that felt me up had contacted the high-risk ovarian cancer center and apparently, they now want to see me every six months because of the cysts that were noted on my uterine lining. Oh boy, how lucky am I? Not only do I get to be "probed" two times a year for the ovarian cancer screening, but I also get it from my regular gynecological visits. I'm thinking at this point there needs to be an entry fee.

I'm off to NYC with my friend Jenna tomorrow. I'm super excited. We are looking forward to a girls' weekend and getting in some quality time with one another because between my life and hers, we don't ever see one another. Though we are going up there to get away, I will also be doing a photoshoot for the SCARProject. I'm excited but nervous at the same time. I will not be doing a full-frontal shot. I would if I could, but I can't, so he will be photographing my lovely back scar.

Monday, October 13, 2008
New York City

My trip to NYC with Jenna was absolutely wonderful. We got into New Jersey sometime in the afternoon on Friday, October 3rd. Since neither of us is very good at making any type of a decision, we had a heck of a time figuring out what we wanted to do– go to the city or stay at the hotel. After a few hours and many back-and-forth of "I don't care," we decided to eat dinner in the hotel and stayed in for the evening to relax and watch a movie. I didn't make it much into the film before I passed out. I think I was asleep by 8:15 pm. I pretty much slept the whole night through, though I woke up here and there while Jenna was watching the movie.

On Saturday, we got up in the morning, had breakfast, and then headed into the city. We took the train over from the airport, which was ridiculously expensive, and I got smashed in the stupid doors as I was entering the train station. I think that is where all of my bruises on my legs came from. We had a bus tour scheduled for 3:00 pm, so we had some time to check out Times Square. We went to Hard Rock Cafe for lunch and then went to Toys R Us to ride the sixty-foot indoor Ferris wheel. It was a great idea at the time, but after the third or fourth time around, we both started getting sick.

We met our tour bus a few minutes before 3:00 pm, and off we went on a five-and-a-half-hour tour of NYC. It was great because we got to see so many things we would never have seen. We went to Central Park, Strawberry Fields (dedicated to John Lennon), John Lennon's residence where he was shot, Rockefeller Center, St. Patrick's Cathedral, Wall Street, Empire State Building, and many, many other places. We went on the ferry from Manhattan to Staten Island and were able to see the Statue of Liberty as the sun was setting. It was gorgeous.

As we were standing on the top deck of the ferry watching Manhattan drifting off into the distance, I decided we needed to have a picture of that moment. As I turned around to see who might be around to take the photo, I saw the most handsome and perfect man in the world right there in front of me. Dear Lord, he was like a twenty on a scale of one to ten. I think my knees went out from under me, he was so hot, and he spoke another language which made him so much more attractive. I literally could not keep my eyes off this man and was so disappointed when out from behind his shadow appeared his girlfriend. Damn! All the good ones are taken. I had contemplated pushing her over the side of the ferry, but she was a bit bigger than me. I would most likely have been the one going over the side. So, I stared at him the entire time to and from Staten Island; awkward, I realize, but I couldn't help myself. I have never seen anyone that handsome. I think his girlfriend was getting a bit nervous because she started "marking her territory." She should have been worried because I was seriously thinking of ways to get rid of her.

We ended our tour at the World Trade Center. It was almost surreal, and I was very emotional. I fought back the tears several times as I stood there looking at the site of where the Twin Towers used to stand and where so many died for reasons that I have never been able to wrap my mind around. Jenna and I went back to the hotel and met my friends Flora and Jeff that were part of the Emerald Dream Ball in Las Vegas. We visited for about an hour and a half and then I had to get to bed.

Jenna and I got up early on Sunday to gather up our things and head over to the city again for the photoshoot. We decided to take our luggage with us instead of going back to the hotel for it. Not a great idea when you have to walk thirty blocks to get to your destination– mostly through Chinatown. Ugh! As we were walking down the street to find a bathroom, we literally brushed against two guys with their kids. I looked at the one guy, who was very good looking, and spun around on my heels as he passed me. I knew him from somewhere but couldn't figure it out. Jenna was behind me and in semi cardiac arrest. It was Ed Burns, the super-hot actor who played George in 27 Dresses. We about peed our pants!! I think he may have realized that we recognized him because he quickly disappeared and was behind some trees.

After calming ourselves enough to continue on our journey, we walked to David Jay's studio. When we got there, the looks of the outside of the building made Jenna a bit nervous. It seemed like she was praying that she wasn't going to get killed. I laughed and said, I hope he isn't hot. As the door opened, there stood a good-looking man with an amazing physique. It was David Jay, the photographer. Damn... I wasn't sure how I was going to handle getting naked in front of this guy. I got my makeup and hair done, and David Jay photographed me for about three hours. At first, I was extremely nervous and stood covering my chest up with my hair and my arms. I have never allowed anyone to see me without my clothes except for my doctors. However, he made me feel very comfortable, and I was able to relax, but I still kept myself covered up. I think I challenged him because I would only allow him to photograph my back, and it took many, many poses to figure out how to get the scar and my face in the photos. I think we finally got something he could work with.

There were two other cancer survivors there while I was doing my shoot. The one thing I noticed about both of them is that they seemed much more accepting of their bodies than I am. They freely walked around without their shirts or bras on, but I tried all I could to hide my body. I wondered how long they have been survivors, and I wondered if I will ever become that comfortable with myself again. Can I learn to accept my body the way it is and to love myself despite all of my imperfections? I don't know the answer to that. I can tell you that right now, I'm not there. I'm actually far from that place.

Jenna and I gathered our things and made the long hike back toward the subway station and then rushed to get to the airport only to have our flight delayed by a half-hour and then again by another hour while sitting on the tarmac.

Overall, it was an awesome experience. I can't wait to go back to NYC. I was totally inspired by David Jay, who is a minimalist. He lives in a studio apartment with only a bed and a table. I loved it. Makes me realize I need to simplify my life much more. I believe the fewer things you have in life, the less you have to worry about it. But as he said, "When you are a minimalist, you must choose things carefully."

Friday, October 17, 2008
Viva Las Vegas

Tomorrow I am headed out to Las Vegas to spend five days with Justin. I haven't seen him since June, and I miss him tremendously. I'm excited yet nervous at the same time. We have some pretty heavy topics that we will need to talk about while I'm out there, and I'm not sure if I'm ready for it.

I suppose my biggest question that needs to be answered is what both of us are looking for through this. I'm not interested in having a long-distance relationship. If I'm going to attempt this relationship thing, I want it to be with someone whom I see on a regular and consistent basis. I don't refer to Justin as my boyfriend, despite my always telling him that I love him, which I do. At this point, he is a person of interest who is geographically undesirable. I'm sure he would like to know that.

After we have the discussion of what we both want out of whatever this thing is we are doing, I need to lay everything out there on the table about all of this cancer bullshit. Justin needs to understand that my body is not what he likely expects it to be. He needs to be willing to accept me in all of my brokenness and not try to fix it because it cannot be fixed. Whether I actually follow through with this or not remains to be seen, but I am taking my cancer journey book to share with him. It is a book that I created for myself to pictorially journal this experience. I have pictures of almost everything in there, from my pre-mastectomy body, all of my surgeries, radiation, skydiving, the Race for the Cure, and many other things. I have never shared this book with anyone, as it is incredibly personal and private. I decided that one day I would use it to show that one special person all that I have been through along my cancer journey. My thinking is that if I show him this book and he decides he cannot handle all of this, he has a way out.

We also need to have a discussion about my not ever having children. I'm not sure where he is on that issue, but he will need to accept the fact that if we are going to share our lives together, it means a life without children. I think this will probably be the hardest thing for me to discuss because I have not come to terms with it as of yet and I'm still very much pissed off by it. But I do feel like I need to get it out there because if he strongly desires to have children, then I know that this is likely where it ends.

I don't know what will happen, and as I said, I don't have very high expectations. I'm mentally preparing myself for the rejection. All of this cancer stuff is a lot to handle. It's not fair to me, and it most certainly is not fair to him. Though I will be very hurt, I can definitely understand if this isn't something he wants.

I know that regardless of how this all pans out, this trip is going to be extremely emotional for me. I'm not sure if I'm ready for all of this. Admittedly, I'm scared as all hell to put myself in a vulnerable position and allow someone on the inside.

Saturday, October 18, 2008
Not What I Had Hoped For

Well, I'm here in Las Vegas and today hasn't been what I had hoped it would be thus far. Really, it has little to do with anything here and more to do with the phone call I got this morning that caught me off guard. My dad called me as I was gathering up my things to put in my car to tell me that my Grandpap Hoberek (my mom's dad) had passed away this morning. I felt like I had been punched in the stomach. I knew that this phone call would be coming sooner than I would like because he had not been doing very well for some time now. I hadn't expected that it would be today.

My conversation with my dad was very brief, and I stood in my kitchen trying to process what he told me. I fell to the floor and cried. I've cried most of the day. I am heartbroken that my Grandpap is gone and I didn't even get the chance to say goodbye. I know that he is in a better place now, and he is no longer suffering. He was to the point where he had dropped a significant amount of weight, was unable to walk, and couldn't care for himself. He apparently had brain cancer but didn't know about that before he passed.

I am obviously not going to the funeral, though I've thought about flying to Michigan so that I can be there. But I feel I would much rather remember my Grandpap the way I last saw him. He and I always had an exceptional bond, no matter the distance between us and I'd rather have that memory than something else. Though it would anger some people by me saying this– I was his favorite. Everyone knew it. Anytime my Grandpap was around, it was almost a for-sure thing that I would be very close by, if not sitting on his lap. I remember being just a little tike and sitting on his lap for hours on end. I didn't want to move, I wanted to be close to him. I used to listen to his heartbeat and try to match my breathing to his. Those are the things I prefer to remember about my Grandpap. He was a very special man to me, and he will be sadly missed. The one thing that breaks my heart the most is that he always wanted to see me get married, and now he will have to see it from heaven.

Friday, October 24, 2008
Life is Hard

Nothing in my life can ever be easy, I swear. Everything about my life completely sucks, but hey, I'm still here, right? Yeah, whatever. I have this black cloud above my head that I can't get rid of, and it impacts all facets of my life. If there is shit to step in, I'm waist-deep. Maybe it's my payback for being such a devious child, I'm not sure.

I'm not ready to talk about anything right now because I'm hurt, confused, pissed off, and a thousand other emotions. The start of my trip to Las Vegas was not a good one with the passing of my Grandpap, but I had a great time while I was there. I got to see some friends, and I was even propositioned by a man because he mistook me for a hooker. I had a great time at Justin's birthday bash, and it was nice to step out of the rat race of life for a few days.

Justin and I never talked; I just wanted to let things happen. I figured that whatever happens, happens. I'm not sure how I can be so smart and so dumb all at the same time. We should have talked, and I deeply regret that we didn't because I'm feeling foolish right now. We had a brief conversation via text message last night that I wish we would've never had. I was left feeling like someone kicked me straight in the stomach, and I want to vomit.

I can honestly say that I'm so fucking tired of life right now and I'm ready to quit fighting. I don't understand it by any means, and I don't get why mine is so particularly hard. Not that I think that anyone's life is all that easy, but I've been waiting for something good to happen to me for about 10 years now. It only continues to get worse. I want it all to stop; I want the pain and the hurt to stop. I would give anything to have one aspect of my life to be tolerable. I know that they say what doesn't kill you only makes you stronger but I'm not that strong, seriously. There are days when I wish it would kill me already so that I don't have to carry around all of this hurt every single day and pretend for everybody that my life is great. Truth is, I hate everything about my life!!!

Saturday, October 25, 2008
Reach to Recovery Mentor

Today I took one of my first steps in working toward achieving my goal of making a difference, changing a life, and touching a heart. After waiting almost a year, I finally completed the Reach to Recovery program through the American Cancer Society (ACS). With Dr. Ahrendt's blessing, I will become a mentor for other women with similar circumstances to mine who are facing breast cancer. I feel like it's one way that I can use this cancer journey positively. I hope that through being able to talk to someone who has been there and does understand, I can make someone else's journey through the cancer world a little more tolerable.

When I called the ACS after I was first diagnosed, the only person that they could link me up with was much older than me, and that didn't seem to make sense. After learning that there were no volunteers my age, that is when I made the decision to become a volunteer myself. Though you technically have to be a year out of treatment, I kind of pushed the issue because I whole-heartedly feel that there is a need for someone my age that other young women can turn to during this experience. I feel good about having gone through the training, and I hope that I gain so much more from being a volunteer than I ever expected.

Monday, November 3, 2008
Celebrating a Milestone and Celebrating a Life

Celebrating a Milestone
Today was my one-year follow up with my radiation oncologist, Dr. Beriwal. He could hardly believe that it has been over a year since I've ended treatment and indicated that he feels like it was only last month that I finished my radiation. I chuckled at him and said, "Trust me. I am well aware that it has been a year since my last radiation treatment." It's hard not to be overly sensitive of time when I have had to go through additional surgeries, expansion, and recovery. He checked my lymph nodes in my armpits and my neck. I hated to say it, but it felt like a massage– bonus (I am so in need of a massage)! He, like all of the other doctors, felt up the foobies, and as always, I wanted to jump right out of my skin. I understand that they need to put some pressure on them to make sure there are no little bastard cancer cells down around my chest wall, but for goodness sake, it downright hurts, at times.

He asked me if I was pleased with the outcome of the implants this time (I had been pretty verbal with everyone about my dissatisfaction with the smaller implants) and for the most part, I am. However, much to my dismay and denial...the right side has dropped from its original position, and I'm not sure what this will mean come Wednesday when I see Dr. Gimbel. UGH!!! Dr. Beriwal also asked about the pain in my back. I explained that it has continued to be present, but it's not constant. Some days are worse than others; I do my best to ignore it. He asked if I was experiencing any other pain to which I had explained that I am not, outside of when people forget how sensitive my frack and my back are and continuously paw on me. I told him that I need to wear a sash that says, "Handle with care" or "Police line-do not cross." He chuckled. I return in exactly one year, November 3, 2009, for a follow-up with him. He smiled when I told him I would put it in my calendar because it's a date.

Since I was down that way, I took my Physician's Approval form for the American Cancer Society up to Dr. Puhalla's office. The secretary was not a very pleasant person this morning, and as much as I wanted to tell her that, I did not. My only concern with that form is the question that asks about me being emotionally stable. I wouldn't be as concerned with this if every time I get one of her reports it didn't say, "continues to experience significant distress related to her cancer diagnosis" and "recommend continued outpatient therapy with a psychologist." We shall see what happens with that one.

Celebrating a Life
Though I was happy to celebrate the milestone of being out of radiation therapy for more than a year now, today was a difficult day emotionally as I mourned the loss and celebrated the life of a very precious little angel

187

who has taught me so much about myself, life, and love through his short time here on earth. My dear friends Kara and Jeff's little Baby Lukey passed away on Thursday at the age of two from a rare disorder. Kara and I formed a bond through our challenging circumstances, and though they are very much different, there are a lot of things that we understand about one another's feelings and what the other has been through. Though I never met Luke, I came to know and love him so very much through Kara's sharing of his journey with me. Luke was such a trooper; his parents are nothing short of angels themselves. The love and care they have given him over the last two years are absolutely remarkable and could be seen in the smile that he always seemed to have on his face. God most certainly knew what he was doing when he picked the two of them to be Luke's mommy and daddy. I have nothing but the utmost respect and admiration for Kara and Jeff as they have handled this situation with such grace throughout, never once complaining about the challenges they had to face or the sacrifices they had to make. I could only wish that there were more people in this world like the two of them. Luke will be sadly missed, but he will never be forgotten.

Wednesday, November 5, 2008
Last Stop. Please Exit the Train!

Well, today was my follow-up visit with Dr. Gimbel, my plastic surgeon, for him to check out the right foobie. I was slightly irritated that I had to sit in the waiting room for almost an hour because they were backed up. Nothing good can come from sitting there for an hour when your head goes a million miles a minute, and you have nothing to distract yourself from all of the thoughts. Finally, I was called back into a room. Dr. Gimbel was in to see me within five minutes. I told him that I had some questions for him and I'm sure he was going to think that I am crazy. I am, but I need to ease my mind by having the answers.

He decided he would take the questions before examining me, which was actually an amusing conversation. I started to ask him, "What type of emergency would warrant my flashing my foobie identification card?" but I only got to the flashing part when he interjected and said, "The implants?" I was laughing so hard I almost peed my pants. I said, "No, that is totally not what I was going to say at all." I finished asking the question, and then he told me that the card I had previously was for my tissue expander and I may have needed it if I set off the metal detector at the airport. Oh! That might have been a good thing to know before I went through the metal detector at the airport with the tissue expanders. Thank goodness it didn't go off because I would have ended up getting stripped searched because that is the last thing I would have thought of. Oh boy! I explained to him that I have had this burning desire to know since someone told me that if I die and they cannot identify my body, they will use my implants. In my head, that didn't seem right by any means. All I could imagine was my charred body with my implants still intact, and I knew that didn't make any sense. He assured me that the purpose of the identification card is not for identifying my body and the foobie identification card does not have the statement "in case of an emergency." I asked him about this "device tracking system" that I had to sign for and wanted to know if there was like a GPS system in my chest. He laughed and said that it's a system for the manufacturers in case something would go wrong. He said, "It's like with cars. Sometimes, ten years down the road, there is a problem with the tail lights or something, and they have to be recalled or replaced." Oh boy. So, now I'm being compared to a car. Hopefully, I didn't get a defective implant. It's bad enough they have to be replaced anyway because they only have a "shelf life" of ten years. That was stupid, I know. I asked him if anyone else complains about the cold and he initially thought I meant that they get cold, which, by the way, is so creepy when I'm working out and nuclear hot, but my foobies are like ice cubes. I have my own personal cooling system. I explained to him that when I'm cold, I have spasms– not fun. He said that no one else has ever complained about that, which I figured as much since I seem to have my own unique set of issues with the implants.

189

He is not surprised though because of my history with the muscle spasms. He asked me what I do to keep them warm, and I told him I stuff hand warmers in my bra. The nurse was concerned that I might burn myself, but I wouldn't feel it anyway.

After entertaining my questions, he checked out his handy-dandy work and is pleased. I pointed out that the right side has dropped some, but he seems to feel the symmetry is still okay with them (riiiigggghhhhhttttt, he isn't the one that is lopsided and has to wear a bra). I asked him if this means I can start running again and he said yes!!! Woo Hoo!! That's super exciting since I need to start training for my first season on the Pink Steel dragon boating team and my high school sweetheart's wonderful and fabulous mother gave me a treadmill! He said I need to be sure that I wear two bras, which I do every day anyway because I'm afraid it's going to fall out at any given point in time. I see it in my head as I'm standing there talking to some super good-looking guy, "Oh, excuse me *bending over*, I seem to have lost my implant." Not going to happen in real life, but it happens in my head, and that's enough to make me wear two bras. I do have to say that when I'm all strapped in like that though, it's not very comfortable. I feel like a Fembot from Austin Powers. They are chicks with machine guns for boobs. They never move without the rest of the body. Odd, I know. But again, this is in my head.

He indicated that the last step would be nipple reconstruction if that is what I want. I have thought about this. Really, they are only for decoration and would serve no other function than hanging Christmas decorations or getting the chained nipple rings, so I'm going without. It's actually cool to be able to wear a strapless top without a bra, and not worry that I look like I'm smuggling Tic-Tacs. I can get tattoos, but I think that would be weird. Again, it would only be for decoration but couldn't hang anything from them. He took some pictures and said that I would need to come back in a year. He said, "Yes, you will be on your own for a year." I looked at him and said, "I love you all dearly, but I have spent way too much time in this office."

I still have a ton of other doctors to see regularly anyway, which reminded me that I need to schedule another who-ha probing. Yippee! Of course, there is a slight catch to the year thing, since the implant on the right side seems to be dropping; I have to keep my eye on it. I'm a slight perfectionist and will monitor that situation closely. He said he has seen women that are as thin as I am experience dropping of the implant, especially if the implants are larger like mine. What? These are hardly large! Anyways, he said that it could be fixed with a simple surgery, which in his head would mean swapping out these implants with smaller implants. In Melissa's head (which will always win), that's a big NO!!! I didn't even get into that conversation, though because it wasn't necessary at the time. As I was leaving the parking lot, the attendant said she hadn't seen me in a while.

Gosh, how pathetic is that– even the parking lot attendant got used to me being there. I told her it might be another year before she sees me there if all goes well.

I got home this evening from work, and the first thing I did was go for my first run, well fast-paced walk. It wasn't as easy as I had hoped it would be because I'm battling being out of shape, an increase in my asthmatic symptoms, and the sensation that I feel in my frack and my back when I run. But it still felt good to get some of my stress out and say fuck you to cancer.

Wednesday, November 26, 2008
The Internal Battle Between Super Bitch and Cancer Fighting Princess

I haven't written in some time, so I figured I should do that...maybe it will help me to get out of this horrible mood that I've been in for a good while now.

First of all, I have to say I've been physically not well for a few weeks. The right side continues to fall, and I've been experiencing excruciating pain in my back and my frack. Saturday was the worst; I was hurting so badly I was on the verge of tears. I lay on the couch for hours, not knowing what to do for myself. The pain has eased up some, but it's still very much there and extremely obnoxious. Add on top of that my emotionally fragile state and you get SUPER BITCH!!!

I think things finally caught up to me this past weekend despite my hardest attempts to keep it all at bay. I finally had some time to think and not do much of anything; I've literally been on the go since August. It hit me all at once, and I've been nothing short of miserable, though no one would know it because I don't show it...thus the battle between Super Bitch and Boobie Cancer Fighting Princess. Super Bitch is only visible when I'm alone. Boobie Cancer Fighting Princess is the little cancer warrior that everyone else sees...she puts on her pink boots with her pink cape, and that big, fake smile every day when she faces the rest of the world. But Super Bitch is a whole other beast that wreaks havoc on my mind, emotions, and soul. How special is it that only I know the real devastation of her?

I'm so unhappy in my life right now, and I don't know what to do to change that for myself. Some of it has to do with cancer, but other things are not related to cancer at all. There are so many things going on that I don't even know where to start. I was so excited to move into my new place, but I've discovered that I hate it here. I would rather be anywhere in the world than have to come here and spend any amount of time. I'm counting down the months until my lease is up and honestly, it can't come soon enough...nine months to go. I would seriously consider breaking my lease, but that will cost me thirteen hundred dollars. I feel like that would be a poor life choice right now with the way the economy is declining, so I'm stuck here for now.

So, my home life sucks. Let's move on. My "love" life– and I use that term loosely– sucks, too. Justin and I have yet to talk, and at this point, I do not believe that we ever will. I'm so completely confused by it all. He is the one who wanted to talk because he was confused about things– like how things were going to work out between us because of the distance between us and where things were going with us. Though I have also been thinking about this, I was less concerned with that. I was blindsided by his response when I sent him a text that read, "I want to make sure that we are on the same page and that you can deal with all the cancer shit, outside of that I'm not worried." His response was something to the effect of yeah, there are your nieces who need you, kids (WTF?), school, doctors, and blah, blah, blah. Nothing caught my attention other than the whole kid thing. It was that word alone that made me feel like I had been kicked in the stomach. Why he was bringing up the kid thing was beyond me because he has known since May that I have no intention of having children. I pretty much broadcasted that to him, everyone in Pittsburgh, and all of my friends when I shared the article from the Pittsburgh Post-Gazette. That has been sitting in the front of my mind for over a month now, with no resolution.

He tells me we will talk, but lately, I don't hear from him. I sent him a text message last night to ask him if he was hating the world or just not talking to me. He said he was fine, so I told him that I'm confused as to why I never hear from him anymore then. He said that he is only talking to certain people right now because he is sorting things out in his life and focusing on the now. He seems to have this issue with talking to anyone when things are not going well in his life. I'm the last person on his list to speak to because as he has said, I am "much worse off" than he is. Through texting, I told him that there is a whole other world of people who love and care for him that he is shutting off from his life. I told him he needs to think about what his shutting those people (me included) off might be doing to his relationships with them. He said he knows. I told him I'm not sure he does, but that is for him to figure out. His response was, "yup," and I replied by telling him I hope he figures it out before it's too late. I ended the conversation there. I have no idea where we stand. I'm baffled; we have no plans to see one another, and if it weren't for me, we wouldn't even talk. I have no idea, but I'm not one to chase after (or sit around waiting for) anyone. I can't emotionally handle someone who shuts me out when things go wrong.

I was asked out on a d-a-t-e (his word, not mine) by a guy I went to college with from my fraternity, and I said yes. Unfortunately, he had to cancel the date, which was supposed to be the Steelers/Cowboys game because he has to be back at Harvard for a presentation and can't get a flight that Sunday. He is coming home this week, and we are going to make plans to get together while he is back in the area. We also talked about hanging out while he is here for Christmas, and I will be in Boston in February for a week, so he has agreed to be my Harvard tour guide while I'm there. I'm looking forward to it because we haven't seen one another for ten years, and it will be nice to be around someone who might actually talk to me.

My home life sucks, my love life sucks, and then there is my social life that almost, like my love life, does not exist. I pretty much do nothing other than work, go to class, and do research for my papers. Gosh, I'm a rock star! I miss being able to drive to Edinboro for the weekend, party with my friends, and not worry about anything other than having a blast. It's hard because most of my friends are engaged, married, and/or have children, and I'm not even remotely close to that stage in my life. I don't fit in anywhere. I can't do dates with my married/engaged friends because I'm the third wheel and who wants to be THAT person, and I don't see any of my single friends because I don't go out to the bars looking to get drunk and find a guy. I'm a lost soul.

All of this leads me to the bigger question that I have been contemplating as of late– what purpose do I have here? I can't seem to come up with one, honestly. My life is pretty empty by all accounts. I'm almost convinced that I'm here for God's entertainment purposes only. I read something that said we experience the "lows" in life to build character in preparation for our eternal life with God. I'm going to say that at this point, I'm full of character– no more need to continue the torturing of Melissa. It can stop now, thank you.

Well, as much as I wish writing all of this would have helped in some way, shape, or form...it has done nothing to shake me out of my Super Bitch mood, so I'm going to watch a movie by myself.

Monday, December 1, 2008
Such is My Life

Mr. Harvard was home for Thanksgiving, and we made plans to see each other Friday night. I was excited to see him and go out to have a good time. I so need it! He texted me earlier in the day asking what I wanted to do for the evening, and since I don't plan and I don't make decisions very well, I gave my standard, "I'm cool with whatever" response. He seemed to like the fact that I wasn't telling him what I wanted to do and said he would devise a plan for us because he is a great decision-maker. Whew! He said he wanted to get a limo for us to cruise around Pittsburgh so that I wouldn't have to drive us. How cute is that? Definitely was a first for me. He asked for a little time to come up with his master plan, and then he would fill me in later. I'm not sure what his plan was, but he wanted to be sure I wasn't overwhelmed by it all and that I was feeling up to it. Well, around 5:30 pm, he sent me a message that his sister went into labor at the mall and was having a baby right at the moment he was texting me. I can't lie, I was disappointed, but I knew he would need to cancel his plans to be with his family and his sister for the arrival of his new nephew. He apologized numerous times, so I know that he was sincere in wanting to see me. He was deployed to Iraq for three years and missed out on many things, so he did need to be there. We plan to get together over Christmas and again while I'm in Boston. So, this episode of my life is to be continued...

My friend Amy from Florida called me on Saturday to tell me that she would be in Pittsburgh with some of her friends and that they would be going out in the South Side and asked if I wanted to join them. I already had plans to meet my friend Denny at Bob's Garage Lounge in Fox Chapel, so I stayed for about an hour or so and then met Amy down in the South Side. I was super excited to be out and about with some of my friends and was looking forward to having a good time. I was okay at first, but as the night continued and everyone but me was getting drunk, I became extremely agitated. With all of the pent-up anger I've had in me as of late, I almost punched some drunk girl in the face because she hit me in the back at least four times. I have never been to that point in my life. I spun around on my heels and had my fist clenched, but then I remembered that she was drunk and it's not like she knew. I had to leave that bar before I seriously hurt someone, so Amy and I separated from the group and went bar hopping for a little while. It was difficult because most of the bars were overcrowded, so the likelihood of my not getting bumped was slim to none. Finally, Amy and I met up with the rest of the group who had gotten a VIP section at one of the bars. It's kind of stupid because you're pretty much caged in from the rest of the crowd. I sat down for a little bit, but then my back and chest started to hurt.

When I couldn't take it any longer, I decided that I needed to leave. I was so angry and frustrated on my drive home because I feel that I should be able to go anywhere that I want and not have to worry about being in a crowded place for fear of getting hit in the chest and in the back. It magnified my awareness of the isolation I have experienced through all of this by about ten times. I wish I could go out, dance, and have fun with my friends without fear of getting hurt. But I can't because the reality is that I have cancer.

Ah, such is my life.

Tuesday, December 2, 2008
University of Pittsburgh's Medical Conference

I got a voice message from Darcy Thull today at work. She is the geneticist that I worked with at Magee when I was first diagnosed and the one to break the news to me that I am indeed a Teenage (and then some) Mutant Ninja Turtle. She called to ask me if I would be a guest speaker for the University of Pittsburgh's annual medical conference on genetic predisposition for cancer. I immediately returned her call and left her a message that I had a few questions but that I would love to be a part of the conference.

The conference is on Tuesday, December 9th from 1:00-3:00 pm at Pitt. There will be at least 150 first-year medical students in attendance. I will share my cancer story with all of them and then answer any questions that they might have for me. I will need to take a half-day off from work to participate in this, but I am excited about it, and I feel like it is another way for me to help increase other's awareness and knowledge of cancer and the genetic mutation.

Saturday, December 13, 2008
Pitt Medical Conference

On Tuesday, December 9th, I shared my story at the University of Pittsburgh. There were two of us there presenting. Since this was my first year, I asked the other lady to go first. She was diagnosed with Familial Adenomatous Polyposis (FAP) in her 40s. Her story was heartbreaking and humorous all at the same time. After she finished and I was ready to share my story, I had to tell the students that my story hardly had the humor that Jeanette's did, which probably had to do with my experience being a little fresher than hers as she was diagnosed in 2002. I also told them that this was my first year doing this, so I was a bit nervous but more than that, I was worried that I was going to cry (and indeed I did: three times). As Darcy was putting up my family tree, I saw something that I was unaware of...my Great Grandmother had gone through a bilateral mastectomy as well. I thought to myself, "so much for advances in medicine" but didn't let that come out of my mouth. I simply indicated that I never knew anything about my great grandmother having breast cancer.

There was a question and answer session following my story. I cried when I was talking about telling my friends and family that I had a definitive diagnosis of cancer. It was especially hard recalling how I shared the news with one of my best friends, Ken. I remember the look of devastation on his face. I didn't even have to say anything, he already knew. He was so hurt, and it was apparent in his eyes. Picturing him standing at my door, trying so hard to hold back those tears, had me doing the same and it tore me apart, right at that moment.

Several students came down to meet me after and thanked me for sharing my story. I must say that I felt so good afterward because I think they all took something away from what I had shared with them. I look forward to doing this again next year and am hopeful for more opportunities to share my story.

Monday, December 22, 2008
Who Says You Can't Go Home?

Well, I have a few things to write about today. I suppose I will start with the fact that I have successfully completed my first semester as a master's level student in the Social Work program at the University of Pittsburgh. I got an A+ and an A in my classes. Honestly, I'm not sure how I pulled that off with everything else I have been doing, but I did it. I'm glad I have one semester under my belt.

As I write this, I am in the process of moving back to my old apartment. I finally decided after four months of living in hell, I can no longer take it there. If I were to remain through the length of my lease, I would likely end up in a mental hospital or worse, at the bottom of a river. There have been multiple things that have occurred since I moved in, and I'd finally had enough. I should have known it was a bad omen when I crashed my car into the side of the garage. Weeks into my new residence, I started having some breathing difficulties. I had been wheezing more and more and realized that I was having a flare-up of asthma. I haven't used an inhaler for years, but it had gotten so bad that I had to call Dr. Andrews, my PCP, for a refill. After spending an extended time in the apartment one weekend, I noticed that there was a black film on my new white computer and when I was blowing my nose, something black was coming out. Gross, I know. When I swiped a few other surfaces, there was black stuff all over the tissues. I called the landlord about it; he seemed to think that it was a waste of money to have the vents cleaned out as the furnace was recently installed. I let it go for a few more weeks and got back in touch with him as it was not getting any better. I had decided that I wanted out of my lease due to health reasons. He didn't seem to care that I have cancer and pretty much suggested that the black stuff in my nose could be coming from anywhere despite my telling him that I had swiped the surfaces. I had gotten a new filter, which seemed to help some, but I was still worried about the black film.

I figured out that this place has zero insulation, so I have literally been freezing my assets off. My body physically cannot handle the cold because the foobies get cold and start to spasm. It sucks. It looks like I'm flexing my pecs, but I'm not (though I can. LOL). I got my heating bill for this past month, and it was over two hundred dollars. UGH! I had been looking at buying a house. I have serious commitment issues, so that isn't a good thing for me to do right now. As luck would have it, I was looking through the online newspaper last Tuesday and saw that my old apartment is still open. I took a chance in calling my previous landlord and asked her to take me back. She very graciously has accepted me back as her tenant and has offered to defer the first two month's rent starting in February as I will have to pay a hefty penalty for breaking the lease. I called the movers, who will be here tomorrow, and set up the date/time for the move. My old landlord sent me the keys in the mail, and I have been moving my things since Thursday of last week. I spent the entire weekend running between the two places and at this point only have a few things left to take over except for the big stuff, which is what the movers will be taking. However, I have everything sitting at the front door for the movers to take out and load into the truck.

My cousin Dennis helped me on Friday, and my friend Cathie helped me on Sunday. She was completely amazed at all that I had done on my own. I have things back up on the walls in the old place, the kitchen is completely put back together, and I shampooed the carpets. She laughed and said, "I have to hand it to you, my friend, when you make your mind up about something, you do it." She is right, and I get that from my Grandpap Hoberek, who passed away in October. I do have to say that despite the cost of getting out of my lease, I have this great sense of relief. It's like a huge weight has been lifted from my shoulders. I finally have a place to go to and call it home. Sadly, I would spend 12 hours on a Saturday or Sunday at work or down at Pitt or anywhere else I could find to avoid being at the duplex. That is no way to live! So, as of tomorrow, I'm going HOME!!!

Saturday, December 27, 2008
Harvard Hot Hands

As of December 23rd, I am back in my old place, and it feels so good to be back home. It is a complete disaster right now, but I'm slowly working on getting it in order. The movers came the morning of the 23rd and were in shock to see that I had almost everything sitting at the front door waiting for them. It took less than two hours to load the truck, drive to my old place, and unload. As much as I wanted to stay to get things organized, I had to go to work. I came home after work and had only a few hours to get some things organized with the help of my friends Cathy and Lauren. They are a true blessing to me.

I then drove out to Burgettstown to have Christmas dinner with my friend Jenna and her family, who are like my second family. I got there late, but they are never on time anyway, so I fit right in with them. I didn't get to stick around for the grab bag, but I trust that Jenna got me something I would like.

I had a d-a-t-e with Mr. Harvard. I picked him up at about 11:00 pm at the Saloon in Mt. Lebanon. It was extremely crowded in there, and I was a bit nervous that someone was going to hit me in the chest or back; I was anxious to get out of there. I didn't know where he was, so I went to the bathroom. When I came out, I started talking to a random guy who was making fun of me for texting and not drinking. As I was standing there talking to him, I saw the secretary from my plastic surgeon's office standing at the bar. Oh, she must have been feeling good because she gave me the biggest hug and kept telling me how I am the best. After a few minutes, Mr. Harvard walked over in my direction and quickly swept me away from my new friends. He took me outside to the smoking area (brilliant, I know). As we stood there talking, I had this uneasy feeling with him. I'm going to go out on a limb here and say that it is because he could have cared less if I talked or walked. I felt like nothing more than an object to him– a prize to be won or a trophy to be mounted on his mantle. I swear he has no idea what my face looks like because he was staring at my chest the whole time. Someone should have taught him that the proper etiquette in attempting to impress a breast cancer survivor is not to make her chest a focal point. All night long, he moved my hair so that he could get a better view of my foobies and did a total body check out several times.

I decided that I needed to leave the Saloon, so we went to Bob's Garage Lounge in Fox Chapel. It was fine, except that Mr. Harvard became Mr. Harvard Hot Hands (H3) and wouldn't stop touching me. You would have sincerely thought that we had been dating for some time rather than being on our first date. Though I kept moving his hands, he seemed to continue pawing at me. Unfortunately, Mr. H3 didn't have a way back home other than me. It was icy out that night, so he ended up having to crash at my place. Yippee. I was humored by the fact that he thought he was going to sleep in my bed. HA! Not a chance on that one. Since my beds were not put together, it was the perfect excuse for him to not sleep in my bed. I grabbed two comforters and made him sleep on the floor. Unfortunately, I had to sleep on the floor with him as I didn't have anywhere to sleep either. He wouldn't stop touching me despite my frequently telling him that I didn't want him to touch me. He was asking stupid questions like, "Do you think I'm attractive?" "Did you have fun tonight?" "Was I checking you out?" He came off as being way too touchy and way too needy for me. He had me so irritated. I wanted to smack him in the head with a shovel when he started telling me that I "want it" because he could see it in my actions and my eyes. I have a hard time with anyone telling me what it is that I want! I was upfront and told him that he wasn't going to get lucky so he might as well not even try.

I told him that I wasn't a floozy pre-cancer and I most certainly am not now. I tried to explain to him that dating and relationships are already hard, and when you add on top of that the whole cancer thing, it is doubly complicated. He said that he could care less about the cancer thing and I'm convinced that is because he would have been content if I hadn't talked at all and would have laid there for him to have his way with me. When he asked me if I was in touch with my sexuality, I almost lost my shit on him. I covered my head with the blankets and stopped talking to him altogether. I can't tell you how happy I was for the morning to come. I got up, took a shower, and then drove his ass home. I think I'm done with the dating thing, after that whole experience.

I went to my parents to celebrate Christmas Eve with my family and my two nieces. It was nice to spend time with my nieces. I wasn't feeling like myself the whole day and was quieter than I usually am. I didn't have much of an appetite, either. I was so out of it that someone was talking to me, and I had no idea at all. I dropped my nieces off at about 9:00 pm and made my way back home. I got through the door a little before 10:00 pm and got ready for bed.

Then it hit me...my stomach started hurting. I wasn't feeling right at all. Soon after, I began vomiting. It was the most violent vomiting I have ever experienced in my entire life. I had stuff coming out from both ends. I was beside myself because I had never been that sick in my life. I was ill until early Christmas morning. Billy, my ex-boyfriend from Erie, had started the drive down here to be with me but couldn't find an open gas station, so I told him to turn around. But I truly appreciated the gesture. I couldn't get off the couch on Christmas day as I felt like I had been hit by a train, so there was no way I was going to do the Christmas thing. My parents drove over to bring me some ginger ale, water, and crackers. I feel bad that they missed Christmas with the family too. I rested for most of the day yesterday and today but am still feeling pretty weak in the stomach. I don't have my appetite back, and I'm convinced that I've lost about 15 pounds. I was to go get my new tattoo today, but I canceled since I'm sure that would make me vomit.

I'd hardly say that I'm ending 2008 the way I had hoped, but I am keeping my fingers crossed for a wonderful start to 2009!

Thursday, January 8, 2009
One Semester Down. Forever to Go

I officially have one semester of my second master's degree completed. I started back to school this week with classes on Tuesday and Wednesday. I'm not overly thrilled with the back-to-back, but there weren't any other options for me at this point. I am taking Research in Social Work and Social Welfare. I can tell that this will be a boring and difficult semester. I'm not so concerned with the Research class as I've had one before and did well, but there is a lot of reading that I have to do for the course. I'm somewhat concerned with the Social Welfare class due to the volume of work (on top of what I have to do for my research class) and the fact that history of any kind is not my strength. Both of my professors seem very passionate about the courses that they are teaching, so I'm hoping that will help. They also are very understanding and are willing to work with me should the need arise. Though I would never use my cancer as a crutch, I do think it is vital for my professors to know what I'm dealing with so that should something come up, they are not taken by surprise. I'm hoping that I won't be overly stressed because I know cancer likes when I'm stressed. I always imagine them in my body with little party hats, and party favors dancing around when I'm stressed, not working out, or doing something else that is not good for my health.

I have an appointment with my gynecological oncologist tomorrow for my six-month check-up. I am glad to go back to Hillman for that instead of Magee as my experience at Magee left me emotionally distraught. I'm hoping to avoid the ovary conversation as I'm still not willing to give them up as of yet and honestly, I don't want to talk about it at this point.

Saturday, January 10, 2009
Six-month Who-Ha Check-up

I had an appointment for my six-month check-up with Dr. Zorn, my gynecological oncologist yesterday, which is by far my least favorite appointment. I got there for my appointment at 12:30 pm and went through the standard weight and blood pressure checks. I was then placed in a room where I waited to be seen for almost thirty minutes. I was slightly annoyed by this because I had changed the appointment to accommodate them, and now, I had to wait to be seen. Finally, the ultrasound technician came to get me and took me into the exam room. I had to empty my bladder before we could start, so she showed me to the restroom and said she would be waiting for me. The passive-aggressive side of me was tempted to make her wait for thirty minutes, but I didn't have time as I was missing work for this appointment. I returned to the room, got changed, and was ready for the probing (well, as ready as anyone can be, I suppose). The tech hadn't even set up yet, so I had to lie there waiting for her...again.

The tech started to ask me questions that she would've known the answers to had she read my chart or even briefly looked at it (one of my huge pet peeves). She asked me if I had breast cancer and as much as I wanted to say, "No, I wear this survivor pin so people will feel bad for me," I didn't. She then said, "Your mother had ovarian cancer, right." I know I looked at her with my, "Are you kidding me?" look and said no, it was my paternal grandmother. It frustrates me to no end when they can't take the time to look at my chart before I come in there. It makes me feel like nothing more than a number. And I also get frustrated when the assumption is that I got the genetic mutation from my mother. Two sets of genes are passed on to every child, not just the genes from the mother. Anyway, after about ten minutes, we finally started and, of all the times I have done this (only two times before), this one was the most painful. I could hardly stand it, and it took almost twenty-five minutes. Then the tech started pushing on my tummy to get a better look. I wanted to scream. I tried to close my eyes and pretend I was lying on the beach with a Red Death in both hands being fanned by my personal cabana boy, Paul Walker, but she kept talking to me. Seriously, it is hard to carry on a conversation with a complete stranger who just happens to be probing your who-ha with some foreign object. As I tried to go back to my beach vacation, I decided that from now on, there will be a fifty dollar entry fee to the who-ha. These are hard economic times, so I'm giving them a break.

I do have to say that I am always humored by the recording of the ovaries because it sounds like a plane flying overhead. For some reason, it makes me giggle.

When we finished, I sat up and looked over at the screen and saw several images marked in red and blue. I wasn't sure what that meant, but I didn't have the chance to look any closer because the tech quickly came over and turned the screen away from me. Surely that wasn't a good sign. I changed and was put back into the room I was in earlier to wait for Dr. Zorn. They had written up a preliminary report (this was new) on the exam, but she would need to talk with me about the results. I was somewhat nervous, but kept thinking to myself- What is the worst that could happen? They could tell me I have cancer? Been there, done that. I'd like something new this time." Well, Dr. Zorn came in a short time later to tell me that I need to continue on the 6-month check-up schedule (yeah, that was my thought in the first place). She showed me the report quickly and said that there were some cysts on my right ovary and then stepped back. She mentioned nothing about the left ovary, which I was more focused on because the tech seemed to spend more time on that side. It had said that the left side is multi-cystic. She said that she is not overly concerned with cancer right now, but I need to monitor my periods over the next 6-months. If things start getting weird, I need to go back in for a biopsy. Depending on the outcome at my next six-month check-up, I may need to do the biopsy anyway. Oh boy, that sounds just great!

As much as I wanted to avoid the conversation, it happened. Dr. Zorn started telling me again that it's recommended I have my ovaries removed after 35 or after natural childbearing years. I think I was rolling my eyes at her because she quickly said, "I'm not telling you what you don't already know, right?" I told her that I think having my ovaries removed is a radical step and that I'm not even willing to consider it at this point in time. I'm still dealing with the breast cancer stuff, and though the possibility of ovarian cancer scares the hell out of me, I am not emotionally ready right now.

After that, I had hoped that my appointment was over, but no such luck. I still had to have my blood drawn for the CA-125 test. I asked to be sure the nurse had a butterfly needle, as she wouldn't be coming near me with any other size. The nurse that drew my blood was excellent and willingly used a butterfly even though we had to fill up six tubes. She initially asked me which arm I prefer she use; I told the nurse that she would need to make that decision because she will be lucky to get a vein. She looked at my left arm, laughed, and said, "I'm not impressed." I laughed and made a point to tell her that I'd warned her that I don't have good veins to be poked as much as I am. She was able to get in on the first try on the right arm, and we sat there for a few minutes filling up the vials. I was grossed out though because I could actually hear the blood coming out. It was like a gurgling noise. It was so gross, and of course, I had forgotten my iPod that day.

My next appointment is on February 10th when I go to see the dermatologist for the full-body skin exam. Yippee!!!!!

Monday, January 19, 2009
Are You Cancer-Free?

I tend to get this question rather frequently and, to be honest, it is a question that I'm asked more often than I would like. I mean no disrespect to anyone who has asked the question because I know that people ask only out of concern for my health and, maybe a small part for their own benefit as well. A few weeks ago, at work on Monday, early in the morning, one of my co-workers questioned me about this whole issue. She had me so darn frustrated that I wanted to scream. I seriously felt like I was on the witness stand, and before I could answer the first question, she was asking me another one. I was trying to be honest with her, which I realize did not necessarily work in my favor. I should have told her what she wanted to hear and been done with it. Instead, it was question after question after question. It started off with, "Are you cancer-free now?" and ended with, "Well, then, are you at least just as normal as the rest of us?"

None of my answers satisfied her questions because she wasn't getting what she was looking for. I'm convinced that she wanted me to say, "Yes, I'm completely cancer-free, and I am all back to normal." Well, that is not the truth, and I believe that unless you want to hear the truth, don't ask the questions. I've not been declared cancer-free. The fact is that none of us are truly "cancer-free" because we all have cancer cells in our bodies, it just so happens that sometimes those little bastards go ape-shit on some of us while others are spared. Outside of that fact, I'm not sure how my doctors would be able to say that I'm cancer-free unless they can conduct x-rays, MRIs, and/or CT or PET Scans through their fingers, which I doubt is likely the case. I've not had any type of scan for well over a year now so unless the cancer cells decide to move their party to one central location (and create a tumor); there is no way of knowing. Yeah, I realize this is likely not the most proactive way for my doctors to approach my situation, particularly since I'm a BRCA2 carrier, but I trust that they know what they are doing. On top of that, I do not think my doctors would ever be so haphazard to use the words cancer-free with me simply because I am a genetic carrier and they know, as I do, that statistically, it is likely to return. I know that my surgical oncologist for one is very careful with not providing me with false hope and I whole-heartedly believe that being told I am cancer-free would do just that. I don't say that to sound negative, but I tend to be more of a realist than anything. I know the reality is that it can come back, so why set myself up for complete devastation all over again by letting my guard down?

In a sense, it is that feeling of not truly knowing that keeps me going– to live life to the fullest each and every day, to take chances on things that I may not have taken chances on before, to love deeply and laugh loudly, and to continue flipping off the grim reaper and defying death. The reality of it is that regardless of whether I ever heard the words cancer-free, it wouldn't change anything for me. The concern of a recurrence would continue to be there each and every day. It doesn't make what I've already been through go away. I'm still very profoundly impacted by all that I have been through during this journey, and I'm not as close to the end of this as I would like to be. I think what most people don't understand is that it never truly ends. For those sitting outside of Planet Cancer, where we survivors live daily, it does seem to stop. Once the surgeries were finished and people perceived me as being "healed," "fixed," or whatever other terms one might want to insert there, the phone calls, emails, and cards stopped. It's as though for most, it no longer exists as an issue. It does not ever end– the hurt, the anger, the pain, the worries, etc. do not go away. I mask them a little better than I have before, but I still have days when I don't want to get out of bed, that I don't want to talk to anyone, that I want to cry and scream, and days when I look at myself in the mirror, I want to smash it. As far as ever being "normal, just like everyone else," I have accepted that I will not be, and my life will not be. I'm learning to live with and accept my new normal, but it is a process. I don't know how anyone can go through all of what I have been through and go back to what it was before.

I recently read a survivor story that was posted on the Young Survivors Coalition website that hit home with me as to why I never want to hear the words "cancer-free." Ultimately, a young woman of 33 was diagnosed with stage 2A breast cancer (like me). Several years later, it ended up metastasizing. She passed away in April 2007.

Thursday, January 22, 2009
Does Anyone Have a Clue??

I called Dr. Zorn's, my gynecological oncologist, office on Tuesday because I'm at a complete loss in understanding what Dr. Zorn meant when she said if my periods (aka Charlie) get weird, I need to go in for a biopsy. I needed a functional definition of the term "weird" because I would think that "irregular" might meet the definition of weird and I definitely am "irregular" (though I know many would argue for the weird part, too). I spoke with the nurse practitioner, who gave me little to no direction of what "weird" means. She said that if I notice any changes in my period, I might want to be seen.

It is always changing. There is no consistency with it at this point; I don't know when Charlie will arrive, how long he will stay, or how much I'm going to get (sounds like a typical man!). Sometimes it scares the hell out of me because it's almost like I'm dying (pleasant visual image, I'm sure). She didn't seem to be too concerned with this because she thinks it is the Tamoxifen. I believe it is Charlie's way of saying FUCK YOU, CANCER!!! He keeps fighting for his right to visit once a month.

The nurse recommended that I go to the gynecologist for my annual pap, at which time they may decide to do a biopsy. For heaven's sake...do I need one? Do I not need one? Are we concerned with the ovaries or are we concerned with the endometrial lining? The only bit of useful information I was able to get from her was that my tumor marker was a 29, which is good, though higher than the last time. Thirty-five is the point where I need to be concerned.

Being the "good" patient that I try to be on most days, I called the gynecologist to schedule an appointment. Apparently, I have not been there since October 2007. Oops...I might have done that on purpose. I'm tired of people shoving foreign objects into my who-ha (and getting no satisfaction from it.). The nurse practitioner I usually see is out of the country right now and apparently isn't willing to come back to do my exam...the nerve! I asked to see the gynecologist that I requested when I started going there, but she is booked until May. Though I'm okay with waiting until May, I decided it might be better to get in sooner. The receptionist asked me if I would like to see Dr. Hugo. I fumbled with my words at this point because I wasn't sure what to say or how to respond. Just the mention of her name made me emotional. This was the doctor who called me at work to give me the news that I had breast cancer- the one I never met. I told the receptionist that in the best interest of the doctor, I would probably not have me seen by her. I am not sure that I would be able to control my tongue enough not to say something to her, and I'm sure I would break down because that was so emotionally traumatizing for me. When I told the receptionist this and explained that

I was beside myself when she called to tell me I have cancer, the receptionist said she remembered that. She shared that everyone in the office was also caught off guard that Dr. Hugo had called me to give me such news and all were unsure of why she did that. I have an appointment on February 11th...the day after my consultation with the dermatologist. Fun, fun stuff!

Since I'm already writing, I might as well include this little bit. I was standing in line to use the restroom last night during our class break. There was a girl behind me who noticed my pin and asked if I was a breast cancer survivor. When I told her that I am a survivor, her reply was, "That's awesome." I know that she meant well, or at least I think she did, but I looked at her and said, "No, not really. I don't think it's awesome." I know I surprised her with my response, but it was one of those things that was in my head and came out of my mouth without even a chance of being filtered. She clarified by saying that it is awesome that I'm a survivor and that I'm still here today to which I agreed, and I thanked her. She followed by saying, "But you look great." I was able to filter the response that was in my head on that one, as I realized I probably already made her feel bad. I said, "Yeah, I'm not what most people envision as a cancer patient or survivor." I wanted to tell her that looks can be deceiving– thus the saying, "Never judge a book by its cover," but I kept that thought to myself. I suppose for most people, it's easier to just look at the cover than to actually read the pages.

Friday, January 30, 2009
Do Ovaries Have Ears?

Just as I began to settle from my gynecological oncologist, Dr. Zorn, recommending I monitor my monthly visits from Charlie for any changes or in her words, "if it becomes weird," and being concerned that I will have to go for a biopsy, things are starting to get weird(er). My monthly visit from Charlie is very irregular as it is, but there are usually two things that are consistent; he comes on a Tuesday around 10:00 am, but never within a specified timeframe like every twenty-eight days. Sometimes he visits every twenty-eight days, thirty-two days, or even thirty-six days. It's always a surprise that I never look forward to. The only other consistent thing about Charlie is that he usually comes in like a lion and out like a lamb and, for the most part, sticks around for about three to five days. Though I never know what Tuesday of the month Charlie will bless me with his presence, I can usually tell when he is about to come by my need to have chocolate pumped straight into my veins. I think I should have an IV drip for it.

I hadn't had a visit from Charlie since before I went to have my who-ha probed at my gynecological oncologist's office, so I'd been waiting patiently for his arrival. I am beginning to think that my ovaries may have been listening in on my conversation with Dr. Zorn because things most certainly have gotten weird— more so than usual. I had anticipated that Charlie would arrive on Tuesday of last week, but he never showed up. Instead, he came on Thursday and wasn't his usual "in like a lion" self. He was only here until late Saturday/early Sunday morning, which is also not like Charlie. I didn't stress too much about that but made a mental note in my head. I thought he was gone and expected that I wouldn't see him until February sometime, but that was not the case. For some reason, Charlie decided to come back for another visit yesterday. I had some symptoms and again felt like I needed a chocolate IV drip. I'm trying not to stress over this, but it scares me. I don't like that she told me to monitor Charlie for any changes and poof, Charlie changes. I want to know what showed up on my ultrasound and sonogram to raise a red flag. I'm torn between calling Dr. Zorn and telling her or letting it go for the moment. There is a part of me that fears that she will say I have to go in for a biopsy. UGH!!! I don't want to do it. I swear, if it isn't one thing with all this cancer bullshit, it is another.

Thursday, February 5, 2009
All is Fair in Love and War. Oh, and Cancer!

One of my favorite sayings throughout my cancer journey has been "Shit happens, wipe your ass and move on." But sometimes, it's not that easy. I've already pretty much written about the most private and sacred parts of my body in my journal except for one– the backdoor– but that changes today. How exciting...a journal entry all about my shit.

I've been experiencing some "symptoms" that have been of concern to me since, oh...I don't know, August 2007. I remember having gone to the bathroom and being stunned and scared shitless (pun definitely intended) that my stool was full of blood– and bright red blood at that. I wasn't sure what to think or do. I'd mentioned it to my dad, but he didn't seem all that concerned with it; we suspected it might have been something related to all the Vicodin I had been on in the previous months. That might have been wishful thinking on my part.

Over the past year and a half, I would say that I've noticed blood in my stool more than a handful of times. Sometimes it is bright red, but sometimes it is black– scary black. However, it is more frequent that there is blood on the toilet paper after I go to the bathroom. That happens a few times per month. Typically, it is associated with bloating, nausea, and pain.

Today was pretty much where I had to draw the line. I was so bloated that I could hardly eat or drink anything. I seriously thought that if I had put anything in my mouth, I might spontaneously combust, despite not having eaten anything. I was nauseated and the pain was severe. My body didn't feel right all day. I couldn't shake the idea that something was seriously wrong. I don't like it when I have that feeling because it is usually true. My mom tells me it is part of my "psychic ability." I was born with a veil over my face, so she thinks I have special powers...too bad my powers aren't to cure cancer!

Against my better judgment, I broke down and called my medical oncologist, Dr. Puhalla. She wasn't around, but I spoke with her nurse. This was, by far, the most awkward conversation I have ever had in my life. It was all about my shit. Your pride goes straight out the window on that one. Anyway, when I told her what had been going on, she was immediately concerned. She was quite disappointed that I have not told any of my doctors about this, ever. I must have forgotten to mention that despite my complete awareness of the association between BRCA2 and colon cancer. Oops! She asked me if I have a gastrointestinal endocrinologist. Dammit!! I knew she was going to say that. I, in fact, do not have one and must admit that I do not want one either. I tried to convince her that waiting a few more months or years to monitor the situation would be fine with me, but she was having no part of that. She said that she would check with Dr. Puhalla but that I need to expect that I will probably have to go in for a colonoscopy. FUCK!!!!!! I don't want to, dammit. I don't want to do it. She said she will call me tomorrow with the date and time of my appointment, which will be with the GI team at Magee.

I'm not going to get myself worked up, or I'll try not to anyway because she did tell me that it could be something like an internal hemorrhoid. Possible, but when I think about the things that cause hemorrhoids, I'm not sure. Low fiber diet, insufficient water, too much lactic acid from dairy products, or a deficiency of vitamin E. I don't have an issue with any of these. There is a part of me that is scared to all hell that it could be something far worse than some stupid-ass (yes again, intended) hemorrhoid. Unfortunately, there is a history of colon cancer in the family of the sperm donor so that little bit of information is sitting in the back of my head taunting me.

I called my friend Jay, a colon cancer survivor, to get some insight on what is going to happen when I go for the colonoscopy. Apparently, the actual procedure is painless because they knock you out, but the prep the night before is pure hell. He said you shit and shit and shit until you can't anymore, and it hurts like hell. WTF!!! This is a bunch of crap, seriously. I don't want to do this, but I'm not sure that I should continue to ignore it any longer. I swear I'm going to have a nervous breakdown over the thoughts of being violated by one more foreign object.

Tuesday, February 10, 2009
Finally, Something Positive!

I went to the dermatologist today for a baseline full-body skin exam. It was relatively uneventful and less intrusive than most of the appointments I have had over the last two years. I wasn't especially fond of the nurse practitioner, but that might have been because I'm not feeling very well, and she was asking me questions that I had already addressed on the information sheet I completed. She even made the comment that she should have read what I wrote before coming to get me...novel idea. Apparently, those sheets are merely for fun, and to make the twenty minutes that you sit in the waiting room go by faster.

After having already annoyed me, she left so that I could get undressed and put the gown on. I had taken my pants off and my ass(ets) were hanging out when she opened the door without any warning. HELLO!!!!!! What happened to knocking??? She likely saw the agitation on my face and started to pull the door shut but then opened it up again. UGH! I grabbed the gown and covered myself for fear of someone seeing my ass(ets). She said, "Don't worry. There isn't anyone out here." Grrr!! That isn't the point, she should have knocked. She asked me some trivial question that most certainly could have waited until I was finished getting into the gown. After all that, I waited about 10 minutes for the dermatologist.

Dr. Margaret Lally, dermatologist, came in, followed by a male resident, and not a hot one, by the way. She asked if the resident could stay for the exam. I looked at her, and she immediately knew that I was not okay with that. I apologized to him and said that I wasn't comfortable with that. I usually don't have much of an issue with that, but this was the first time that my entire body from head to toe would be examined. The exam itself was pretty quick, starting with the front and then the back. She noticed the scar on my back and asked what they had done to me. I explained that they took my latissimus muscle. She seemed shocked when she asked how much of it, and I said all of it. She then asked me what I have back there for strength, to which I replied nothing. She wanted to know if I could tell the difference. Yes. Everyday. Dr. Lally said that my skin looks good and there wasn't anything of concern so I will only need to return if something becomes a concern. YAY! Although I was not too concerned that she would find anything.

She recommended that I get a Vitamin D deficiency test because new literature suggests that there is a link between breast, ovarian, and colon cancers and a deficient level of Vitamin D. I was stunned when she said that because no one has ever brought that up to me before. Apparently, some oncologists buy into this, and some do not, thus the reason it is not the standard operating procedure to have the blood test done. However, it may become mandatory in the future. What they have found is low levels of Vitamin D in breast, ovarian, colon, and melanoma patients specifically in the northern climates and a higher incidence of these cancers in this area. Who knew? Not me! If I am deficient, I'm saying BRING ON THE SUN!!! I love the sun, which is how we get Vitamin D for the most part. She said that I would simply need to take a pill to increase my levels of Vitamin D. Easy enough for me! I will have the blood test done at Magee on March 9th when I go for my colonoscopy because there is one guy, Chris, that gets me on the first try, and he willingly uses a butterfly.

I go to the gynecologist tomorrow. I must admit that I'm a bit on edge about this appointment, especially since Charlie decided to show up again this week. He has been here three times in the last four weeks; very unusual for him. My body hates me much more than usual lately.

Wednesday, February 11, 2009
Why Does My Body Hate Me So?

I'm not in the mood to write this journal entry, but I need to express myself and my frustration somehow. I went to the gynecologist today at the recommendation of my gynecological oncologist because my period, in fact, has gotten "weird" and, in all honesty, I haven't been for an annual check-up since October 2007, so I was well overdue. I had a period on January 22th and another on the 29th and then again on February 9th. That definitely constitutes weird, I think.

The gynecologist that I met with was not my usual doctor, which meant I had to go through the whole process of explaining my story. She seemed to be extremely frustrated with me because I couldn't give her exact dates of my periods over the past six months. Who the hell keeps that information in their head? I was agitated with her when she told me, "Well, the first thing we need to do is get you to start tracking your periods." Well, I already do that, but it's on a calendar at home that doesn't fit in my purse. I'm not completely stupid. It's the only way I would have any idea of when I might expect to see Charlie since I went off the pill in March 2007. She then asked me what I was doing for protection. She automatically assumes I'm having sex? I told her that I was abstaining, and she said well, we need to think of some other options but wanted to be sure I couldn't be pregnant. What? Um, NO! I told her that I'm abstaining because I am not in a relationship at this point, and even if I were in a relationship, it wouldn't mean I would be having sex. If I were having sex, then I would be using a condom. I seriously wanted to bang my head off the wall. Why do we need to talk about me having sex when I'm NOT having sex???

Anyway, she did the exam, and I knew something wasn't right because of the amount of pain I had when she was pressing on my left ovary. I knew that she was going to tell me what I did not want to hear– I have to go for more probing. How did I get so lucky? She said there is what appears to be a 5cm cyst on my left ovary. She isn't sure if it is a cyst or something else, so I have to go back for another ultrasound and sonogram (I recently had one done January 9th). She said that from those tests, it would determine if I need to have an endometrial biopsy or have a D&C (dilation and curettage), which would consist of them opening up my cervix and taking a closer look to see what is going on. At that point, I seriously wanted to curl up into a ball and cry like a baby. I'm tired! I'm so fucking tired of all of this.

I have to go on March 6th to have my who-ha probed, and then I go on March 9th to have my backdoor probed. I decided that I'm getting tattoos above both that say, "EXIT ONLY." Of course, this conversation about my current situation with my ovaries led to the conversation that I hate having, "You need to start thinking about when you have had enough of this and just have your ovaries removed." No! No! No! I am not doing that right now. Actually, I don't want to do it ever. I'm tired of my body being hacked apart and them taking pieces of me. She recommended that I make an appointment within a week after I have my ultrasound/sonogram. I'm assuming she got the memo that says, "Don't call at work to give bad news." Good for her.

So, here I am- numb and sick to my stomach over all of this. Granted, it could be nothing, or it could be something. We can't know until the test results come back. I have had numerous, well-intentioned people talk to me about several things regarding the most recent events. I understand that going in for some of these tests may not be all that bad for some people, but when you have gone through it as much as I have recently, it is tiring and monotonous. It is wearing me thin. I'm not sure how much more I can carry on my shoulders. Granted, I am happy that I'm still alive and I do whole-heartedly cherish every day, but when do I get a break? What the hell did I do to deserve all of this? The armor that I have worn over the past two years is getting heavy, and I'm constantly being knocked to my knees. Getting back up continues to get harder and harder.

I'm SICK AND TIRED OF BEING SICK AND TIRED!!!!!!!!!!

Thursday, February 12, 2009
Heaviness in My Heart

After much thought last night, I decided that I don't want to go to the High-Risk Ovarian Cancer program at Hillman to have another sonogram and ultrasound done. Since it will be the gynecologist that makes the decision for the next step, it seemed silly. I am instead going to St. Margaret, which is five minutes from work and home, to have the tests done. I will go on March 2nd for the tests, and then I see the gynecologist on March 10th. Today, I'm much better emotionally than I was yesterday, but I'm still fairly pissed off at the world. My heart is so heavy with hurt and anger, even though I know it could be nothing because I also know it could be something.

With the recent turn of events, I've been very hesitant to plan my second cancerversary celebration for fear that the party meant to celebrate happiness and triumph would only become a pity party for me. However, I have decided that I am going to celebrate my 2-year cancerversary because I deserve it and I need it. This year it falls on a Sunday, which is better than Saturday since St. Patrick's Day happens to be the second craziest time in the city of Pittsburgh, right after the Super Bowl parade.

Tuesday, February 17, 2009
Harsh Reminder

I got a voicemail at work this morning from Kristen, the nurse at Hillman, to call her regarding my appointment for the pelvic exam. I knew what she was going to tell me before I even talked to her. I called her and then she called me back. Since I have been going to Magee for all of this silly business with the BRCA2 mutation, it is recommended that I go down to Magee for the exam instead of doing it at St. Margaret. I whined to her that I don't want to go to Magee, but she insisted and said that even Hillman was not an option–it has to be Magee. She said that if I have it done at St. Margaret's they will just send it to Magee, and I will have to have it repeated. GRRRR!!!!!!

My appointment has been rescheduled again to February 23rd, which is the day I leave for Boston. The last experience I had at Magee was in July 2008 when my appointment at Hillman got mixed up. I swore I would never go back there again. As I've learned, there isn't much in my world that is within my control. I can't emotionally handle seeing all the pregnant women because that will never be my reality. It's a harsh reminder, a punch you in the face kind of thing, that my dreams to have children have been crushed because of stupid cancer. UGH! Stupid cancer! I hate stupid cancer! I will see the gynecologist on March 4th as a follow-up to my appointment on the 23rd.

I have to go to my primary care physician, Dr. Andrews, today because I have been sick for thirteen days now and can't shake whatever it is that I have. I feel like I've been run over by a train. I have not been this lethargic since I went through radiation. I'm completely wiped out, and I have a research paper due today and a mid-term tomorrow.

And of course, because my luck sucks and there can't be any glimmer of hope for me in any realm of my life...

I did have a date on Valentine's Day. I know! I said I was done! All things considered, it went very well, and he didn't paw at me like my last date did. We actually had a great time together and hit it off very well, but there is one small problem...his age. For heaven's sake he is 22 years old...soon to be 23 (on the 23rd). Yeah, should have asked that question before I agreed to go out with him *mental note to self*. I'd be lying if I said that I'm not attracted to him. I am (and have been since I first saw him months ago) and I've been waiting for him to ask for my phone number. He seems to think that he would like to see me again and does not care that I'm *uh hem* old(er) or that I have cancer. Very sweet on his part, but even if age were not a factor, the cancer is a huge issue. I couldn't even think about putting something so heavy on someone so young. It is sad, really. He is one of the very few genuine guys interested in ME in years. Such is my life...

Friday, February 20, 2009
Two-Year Milestone

Well, today makes it two years since I discovered the lump in my boobie. It's almost surreal when I think about the whole thing. I can hardly believe that I have been through all that I have in the last two years and most days, continue to find a way to smile. It most certainly was a very defining day in the life of the person I have become over the past two years. So many emotions are involved in this day. There is still a lack of understanding of how my own body could betray me so much, but there is also great joy at the same time that for whatever reason at that very moment on that very day, I happened to touch that exact spot to find it. There are a lot "what ifs" that have spun around my head at times. For as much as I don't understand all of this, and most likely never will, I am thankful that two years later, I'm able to sit here and write in my journal.

And of course, it goes without saying, but I need to say it...it also reminds me that I have been surrounded and continue to be surrounded by so much love throughout this journey. I know that will continue as I venture around the next corner, regardless of the outcome. I know that I am loved so much even without words, but I did get a message from someone very dear to my heart who knows the significance of this day as a little reminder of the great love that surrounds me. (Thanks BFF, and Happy Birthday! Love u!) Words can hardly even begin to express the depth of gratitude I have had every day for the past two years for all of those that love and care for me.

Monday, March 2, 2009
Ultrasound/Sonogram

I went for my ultrasound/sonogram on February 23rd to follow-up on the 5cm cyst on my left ovary. I'd been dreading the appointment because the whole experience is emotionally taxing for me. I arrived for my 1:30 pm appointment and as I suspected, the place with packed with pregnant women. I stood patiently in line waiting to be checked in and to get the form that I needed to complete all the while thinking that I'd rather be eating glass. The receptionist indicated that they were two hours behind schedule and handed me a pager. I know the look that came across my face was one of pure disgust. I explained that I didn't have two hours to wait because I had a flight to catch to Boston. She then asked me if I wanted to reschedule. For one of the very few times in my life, I stumbled over my words, which was probably a good thing because the thought in my head was "No, I don't want to fucking reschedule." I incoherently rambled something about my doctor that I'm sure made no sense to anyone. I know she could tell that I was extremely frustrated so she quickly disappeared and then returned to tell me that the techs will do the best they can to get me in.

With all the spare time I thought I would have, I decided to make my way down to the lab to have my blood drawn for the Vitamin D deficiency test. That apparently isn't a test that is done all that often in the lab because Chris (my favorite) had no idea what needed to be done. For some reason, having my blood drawn hurt more than usual, even with the use of a butterfly and I bruised pretty bad after. The bruise has finally started to go away.

As I was finishing up with Chris, my pager went off. SAWEET!!!!! The tech indicated that since I'd recently had the ultrasound, she was not going to repeat that so I would only be doing the internal sonogram. I liked that I had a screen right in front of me so that I could see what she was looking at. Sure enough, there was a huge mass on the left side. I was definitely taken back by the size of it. It looked like a plum and then some. I was freaked out when she switched over to the right side, and I saw that the ovary on that side looked to be a little smaller than a walnut. She didn't seem all that concerned with it, but I've come to learn that I can't trust that alone. I was there for only about twenty minutes and then gone. With the exception of the initial waiting to get checked in, it wasn't all that bad, but it still most certainly isn't high on my list of favorite things to do. She made some comment to me about not having to come back to see her and I chuckled to myself. I won't see her, but I will go through the same course of tests in July. I go to see the gynecologist on Wednesday as a follow-up to this appointment. I suppose I will have to wait to see what she says.

So, Boy (my Valentine's Day date) and I have been hanging out as often as I can manage. I have seen him about four times since we first went out, and he is always eager to know when he can see me again. I'm still hesitant about his age. I have expressed that concern to him. I've don't believe or think it is fair for someone his age to have to deal with me and my cancer, but he continues to ignore me in that regard. He is super sweet, and I have teased him about having purchased the "Melissa Manual" off eBay or Craig's List because he always seems to have the right response for everything. He came over last night, and my intention was to go to Funfest to play some video games and of course, subject him to Dance, Dance Revolution, but as luck would have it, my cold has returned. WTF??? He asked to hang out with me anyway, so I agreed. Boy made me homemade vegetable soup and brought me some mineral bath. He is the cutest thing ever, seriously. I'm pretty much beside myself because there is a part of me that wants to push him away because I think he is too young, but then there is a side of me that truly enjoys his company. For the first time in a long time, he makes me feel like I'm second to none. Unlike my ex-boyfriends that tend to pop in and out of my life when they have ended a relationship with another girl. I've always been the "Well, if things don't work out, I'm coming back for you" girl...not by my own choosing. This guy is absolutely nuts about me. Though I can't figure out why, I'm going to go with it and see what happens, or at least I'm going to try.

Thursday, March 5, 2009
Ultrasound Results

I had my follow-up appointment with my gynecologist yesterday to go over the results of the ultrasound. I waited in the room for almost forty-five minutes before she came in, so I listened to my iPod and took a nap. She indicated that I do have a 5cm cyst on my left ovary. Yup, I knew that; I saw it with my own two little peepers. However, she indicated that it does not look to be anything of concern, so she is not recommending a biopsy or a D&C unless I feel like I need that reassurance. Nope, I'm all good on that end, thank you. She asked that I continue to monitor my periods, which at this point, I have not had anything since February 9th. If I start to have irregular bleeding again, I need to go back into see her and as she said, "We will need to figure out what you are going to do to take care of this issue," meaning have the ovaries removed. I'm not sure why everyone seems so obsessed with getting my ovaries out of my body. I looked at her and smiled while thinking to myself- there is no way that I'm having my ovaries removed...not today, not tomorrow, and not anytime in the near or distant future. If all goes well with my periods *crossing fingers* then I won't have to go back for another year to see her. Of course, I do have to go back in July for the ovarian cancer screenings with my gynecological oncologist, Dr. Zorn. I hope that I will not have to go back to the regular gynecologist, and by this time next year, Denise, the nurse practitioner, will be back. I like her much better. I'm relieved that this test didn't reveal any type of malignancy or, anything to indicate that it could possibly be malignant. I am a bit nervous about the upcoming test on Monday, but I'm trying hard not to think about it. I don't know who will be in touch with me regarding the results of that test, but I assume that if there is something of concern, I will be notified rather quickly. I imagine that by Saturday or Sunday, I will be a big ball of stress.

Friday, March 13, 2009
Pooper Probing

I had the colonoscopy on Monday. The actual "pooper probing" wasn't as bad because I was knocked out, so I never even knew it happened. I was a bit creeped out that I saw and talked to the doctor prior to him performing the procedure. I felt like he should have at least taken me out for dinner or something first. The worst part of the whole thing was that I was starving and didn't leave the apartment much over three days. The prep wasn't even that bad. Apparently, I'm not as "full of shit" as everyone tells me I am. I wasn't able to eat anything all day Sunday or Monday, and my appointment wasn't until 4 pm. I tried to tell the nurse on Friday that it's not very nice to starve the skinny kid, but she seemed to think it was a necessity.

My friend, also my ex-boyfriend of five and a half years, Billy, came down from Erie to take me to my appointment. He is attempting to earn the co-survivor title that my BFF, Ken, has earned. I appreciate Billy's efforts but I'm pretty sure that Ken isn't willing to give up his title for the ex-boyfriend or anyone else, for that matter. Anyway, Billy did a great job taking care of me and actually helped out with cleaning the apartment (it's like a tornado comes through when he visits). He even changed my sheets on my bed for me.

He seemed a little beside himself when we were in the pre-op room. I don't think he knew what to do when I started crying and asked him to hold my hand when the nurse inserted the IV. He held my hand, but he seemed to get all choked up over the sight of me being in tears. He didn't stay to take me home, as he had to make his way back to Erie, so Annette came to take his place. I came out of the anesthesia much faster than usual, but I'm sure it was because it was only a twilight. I was still agitated with the nurse, as usual, for waking me up, but as soon as I got into step-down, I put my clothes on and was out the door.

Annette spent the night with me to be sure everything went okay. I woke up the next morning feeling a bit weak in my stomach (could have been the Burger King I ate– it was a necessity...) and was somewhat out of sorts. I wasn't able to go to work on Tuesday since it is illegal to drive within twenty-four hours of having anesthesia. I was finally able to drive around 6, so I went to the Living with Cancer in Your 20s and 30s group at Gilda's Club. It's always good for my soul to know that I'm not going through this alone.

I don't know the results of the colonoscopy as of yet. The doctor said he didn't see any signs of cancer, but I was told to call in two weeks for the results of the biopsy.

224

I finally got the results of my Vitamin D deficiency test. To my, and everyone else's, surprise, I am NOT vitamin D deficient. I was shocked by this as most people do have a deficiency. I'm not exactly sure how it is that I'm getting enough. I suppose it only proves that your genetic make-up trumps the other things that one can do to minimize the development of cancer. It only supports my theory it doesn't matter what I do to try to prevent this from happening all over again; if cancer decides to go ape-shit on my body, then it will do just that. But it also leaves me wondering (still) why my body would betray me, but the biological sperm donor that passed these genes onto me has not had his body betray him.

Monday, March 16, 2009
Two-Year Cancerversary Party

Yesterday I celebrated my 2-year Cancerversary with my family and friends at the Pleasure Bar. Though my friend Chris and I were late getting there because we had been out the night before partying like the rock stars we know we are, I think everyone had a wonderful time. The food was great, I'm sure. But I didn't get to eat because I was chasing my nieces around and well, I can't ever stop long enough to eat when they are around. I wouldn't change that for anything. It was great to see all of my "worlds" collide at one time and almost all in pink. I wanted everyone to know how I was feeling because I'm not always very good with sharing my thoughts and feelings outside of this forum, so I took some time to write something from my heart that I shared at my celebration. I shared how hard the past few years have been for me but having so many people surrounding me through has been a true blessing.

I also made the announcement that after much long thought and prayers, I have decided that I will not be returning to Pitt after this semester. The time demands have been more than I can handle and will only increase over the next three years. I've started to lose sight of what my priorities are, and school has virtually consumed my life. When the grim reaper is banging on your doorstep every day with his Adidas shoes on and a boom box in his hand, waiting to have a dance-off with you in the morning, you start rethinking things. I decided that if I should one day lose my morning dance-off with death, I would much rather have spent my time being with my friends and family and living life than sitting in a classroom. All is not lost in the year I spent at Pitt though, I have gained much more...I have a wonderful new friend I hope will be a part of my life for a long time to come.

Sunday, March 22, 2009
Life is so Unfair...

My Uncle John (my mom's half-brother) came to visit this weekend from Michigan. It was the first time I have seen him in ten years or so, and the first time I have seen him since we both were diagnosed with cancer. I talked to my mom earlier in the morning and cried afterward because I wasn't ready to see my uncle...not this way, anyway. Though it took everything in me not to cry when I saw him, I didn't because I didn't want to make him feel any worse than what I imagine he already does. He is only 44 years old but looks much older. Cancer, radiation, and chemotherapy have obviously taken their toll on him. I never imagined that at any point in our lives we would be sitting around talking about each of our experiences with cancer. I never imagined that I would be staring in the face of my uncle at the age of 44 and watching cancer suck the life right out of him. That was so hard and so not fair.

I got to meet his new wife Lynette and his two precious little ones, Robert (3) and Loren (4). The kids absolutely adored me. They were the cutest things ever and couldn't get enough of me. I took them to the park for a little bit to give my Uncle John and Lynette a rest and to allow my mom and uncle some time to visit. The whole time we were at the park, a billion thoughts were running through my head. I wanted to hug those kids and cry knowing their dad will not see them grow up. I wanted so desperately to hold on to them and to protect them from this evil thing that will eventually take their father away from them. He tells them that one day he will be waving to them from the moon, and it saddens my heart because I know that it's true. They have no understanding that it means their dad will no longer be here with them– to hug them every day, to say, "I love you," and to be the wonderful father that he is. I imagined how each of them would feel as they reach significant milestones in their lives, without their father there to encourage and cheer them on. Gosh, it tore my heart to pieces. I don't understand it, and I know that I never will, but I keep pleading with God to please let him stay. Don't take him away from his family, and, most of all, his children.

After spending about four hours with my uncle and his family, I had to make my way back to my place to write a paper I had blown off so that I could see him (well worth it). As we said goodbye, it felt like a knife was cutting straight through my heart. I didn't want to let him go because I didn't know if this would be the last time I would see him. I wanted to tell him that I wished it were me instead. I would gladly take his place if it meant I could spare his life so he could see his babies grow up, but none of that ever came out of my mouth. I cried the whole way home with so many memories and thoughts running through my head, all the while begging God not to take him and bargaining with Him that if a life must be taken, take mine instead. I can't even bear the thoughts of those kids growing up without their father. It is so unfair!

Friday, March 27, 2009
All Clear

I called Dr. Steven Abo's office on Monday to get the results of the biopsy as directed by the recovery room nurse on the day of my colonoscopy, but only got the nurse's voicemail. She called me back and left me a message to indicate that no biopsy had been done (whew...that had me a bit worried. Not sure why the nurse had told me that in the first place but, whatever) and that the results of the colonoscopy showed no signs of cancer. YAY!!!!! She recommended I go back in for another colonoscopy in 5-10 years. Sure thing, I will get right on that...March 9, 2019.

She didn't tell me if they had found anything that would explain the issues I have been experiencing, which was not comforting. They don't know what is causing it, which means I don't know either. At this point, I only know it happens and sometimes I hurt like hell from the pain. It's like the unexplained back pain that I still have, and NO, it is not old age! Oh well, I suppose it will be left as one of those mysteries of my life. I have an appointment to see my medical oncologist on April 8th. I see my surgical oncologist on May 5th. I'm looking forward to June being a month of no doctor appointments. And, I'm crossing my fingers for a free trip to Missoula, Montana for a week.

I must admit that I'm feeling good about my decision not to continue at Pitt after this semester. A few other things have presented themselves to me, and I'm excited to take on the challenge. First of all, my research professor wants to meet with me after the semester to talk about some options that she feels might better suit me and fall in line with my life priorities. She has repeatedly told me that my work is worthy of a doctoral-level program, and she has some schools in mind for me. It's not that I don't like school; I do. I love being in the classroom and learning, but I don't feel like this program is the right one for me.

Also, through the encouragement of one of my fellow cancer cronies, I am now one of the "Faces of Gilda's Club." It is an initiative to increase awareness of cancer in young adults. I'm not sure how many of us there will be, but we will be involved in several events and activities throughout the spring and summer. We will be featured in the Pittsburgh Magazine, and they are working on getting KDKA and WTAE involved as well. I'm pretty excited about all of this because I have always pushed the need to increase awareness, which is why I wear my survivor pin every single day and proudly display that I am a cancer survivor. There will be a kick-off for the event on April 4th, and the event will end with a comedy show on September 17th called "Laughing in the Face of Cancer." As part of my accepting the nomination as one of the faces, I have set a personal goal of raising $2000 to be donated to Gilda's Club, so I will be pretty busy this summer with hosting and attending fundraising events. In addition to

228

that, I am planning to finally jump on board with the Pink Steel Dragon Boating team, which is something I've wanted to do for some time but couldn't because I didn't have clearance from my doctors. I'm also planning to become more involved in my volunteering efforts with the agencies I currently work with.

All in all, I think it was the right decision for me. I feel positive about things in my life. I must admit that my happiness is also in part influenced by Boy. We have continued to see one another, and he makes me feel amazing– alive and amazing. We are not an item at this point, and I don't yet know if that will happen. I'm simply living in the moment and enjoying the time I have with him.

And on a final note, I will be included in a new breast cancer book geared toward young women. I don't know the release of the book but will be getting a copy of it for sharing my story with the author.

Hmm...and I thought I needed a piece of paper to tell me I would be good at working with and advocating for other cancer survivors. Silly me!!!

Tuesday, April 7, 2009
Today's Faces of Gilda's Club

April 5th through April 11th is Young Adult Cancer Awareness Week. With this week being an important one for me and all of my 20s and 30s cancer cronies, Gilda's Club held the official event kick-off for Today's Faces of Gilda's Club on April 4th. I must say that for the slight coercion it took on the part of my friend, Jay, to convince me to do it, I am happy that I did. I wasn't sure what it actually involved or that I would have time for it, but since school is done on April 22nd, I will have a lot of spare time on my hands to raise two thousand dollars toward Gilda's Club. Actually, I have already started the fundraising process. Both of my schools have agreed to do a "jeans day" in which everyone can pay five dollars toward my fundraising efforts for permission to wear jeans that day. I was able to hand over two hundred-seventy dollars on Saturday, and that was from only one of my two schools! One of my teacher friends is willing to do a fundraiser for me at her restaurant.

The event on Saturday was a great turn out. I'm not sure how many "faces" there are, but I know the goal is to get 50. The faces are survivors, oncology professionals, and friends and family of cancer survivors. As one the "faces," I am not only charged with raising money, but also to increase awareness of cancer in young adults and spread the word about Gilda's Club and the support and services that it provides free of charge to anyone touched by cancer. We are also charged with having fun while we are raising the money. I'm pretty sure I can easily handle that one. All of the nominees were introduced at the event, and we were photographed by the Pittsburgh Magazine. I believe there will be an 8-page spread on us in the June issue.

On Sunday, I went down to the Improv in the Waterfront to be an extra in the commercial for the culminating event to be held on September 17th called Laughing in the Face of Cancer. We were there for approximately five hours filming for a thirty-second commercial. It was fun, but the bright lights ended up giving me a headache. Who said fame was easy? The commercial is expected to be up within a month on YouTube and will be titled Laughing in the Face of Cancer.

After the events on Saturday and Sunday, I realized that it's crucial for me to do this. I am always trying to find ways to get my face and story out there so that maybe, maybe, it will help someone else through their cancer journey. And I'm always looking for ways to increase awareness that this disease can (and does) impact young adults. I also realized the importance for me to do this because I often think about the legacy I will leave behind. Since I will not be having children, mine will be different than most. I guess turning something so negative, devastating, and life-changing into something positive is the legacy I hope to leave behind when I'm no longer a part of this world.

230

Tuesday, April 7, 2009
Don't Ask the Question if You Don't Want to Know the Answer

I went to see my medical oncologist, Dr. Puhalla, today for my routine three-month follow-up. I was there for about an hour and a half but didn't mind as it gave me time to read an article for class and to take a quick catnap. I saw three people today, which isn't typically the case. The nurse practitioner was the first one to see me. Apparently, she is also the nurse practitioner for my gynecological oncologist, Dr. Zorn. I can't say I remember her, as I try to block out those appointments. Anyway, she simply checked my vitals and asked a few questions. I was okay with everything except for when she was checking my breathing. For some reason, I had a feeling she was going to put the stethoscope right on my scar, and damn if she didn't. I know she didn't intend to do it, but it made me jump because it is still so sensitive. Instead of moving it, she continued to press it up against my scar until I finally told her that she was on my scar and needed to move the stethoscope. Mental note for next appointment: make sure the person checking my breathing is aware of the scar on my back.

She left, and shortly after that, the research coordinator came in to say hello. I was nervous at first because I thought for sure she was going to ask to get some blood. She asked me when I would be having my next mammogram...HA-HA...never. She said that women who have gone through reconstruction have an MRI every year. I explained to her that I have only had one MRI, which was done on March 21, 2007. She thought I should bring it up to my medical oncologist (right...like I want more tests). She further explained that there have been changes in the research study that I'm a part of...there is no blood work, or MRIs needed any longer. They simply ask you how you are feeling, and that's the extent of it. She left, and I was able to take a quick nap again.

Dr. Puhalla came in and we chatted about life for a bit. She was sad to hear I am leaving the program at Pitt but understood my rationale for it. Dr. Puhalla seemed a bit concerned that the GI doctor hadn't found anything at all in doing the colonoscopy and then became exceptionally concerned when I told her that I again had symptoms the other day. She wants to get in touch with the GI doctor and ask him if we should conduct an upper scope because of the symptoms that I described and obviously because of the BRCA2 mutation, which makes any and all cancers fair-game. She said that she would have someone from the office call me to let me know if and when I will need to go in for the scope. OH YAY!!!! Exactly what I wanted...more tests. But I suppose, if there is something to be found out by doing it, then I'd rather go through the process of more testing. I had asked her about the MRI, but she didn't seem to think that was necessary and I'm cool with not having to do another one.

I asked her the question I thought I already knew the answer to in my head, but never had the nerve to ask. I suppose it was better to have simply left it known in my head and not hear it come out of Dr. Puhalla's mouth. Numerous people have been asking me if the cancer is gone and my only response to that is, "I don't know" and then they usually ask, "Well, don't your doctors know?"

My response to that is, "I don't think they do, and I'm not sure how they would know." I was right. I asked Dr. Puhalla if she knew that the cancer is gone...NOPE. UGH. That was definitely a blow even though I'd known it all along. Then I asked her, "How can we know if it is gone?", to which she responded, "We can't." That made my day. There is a lesson to be learned here: if you don't want to know the answer to the question, then don't ask. I'm definitely making a mental note on that one.

I go to see my surgical oncologist, Dr. Ahrendt, in May for my one-year follow-up. I suppose I will wait patiently to see what the outcome is regarding the need for an upper scope.

Friday, April 10, 2009
Upper Endoscopy

At Dr. Puhalla's suggestion, I scheduled the upper endoscopy yesterday. I will be going in on April 27th for the procedure. I will have to be put under again, and they will put a camera down my throat to see if they can figure out why I'm having the symptoms that I continue to have. I'm crossing my fingers that they figure out what the issue is, and we can deal with it, whatever it may be. The conversation with the receptionist was rather humorous when I called to schedule the appointment. At the start of the conversation, she was asking me some identifying questions so that she could locate me in the computer. Once she found me this is what she said, "Melissa Ward, history of breast cancer, bilateral mastectomy, rectal bleeding." Seriously, really? That is how you are describing me? Come on. I've often thought I should come with a label describing the contents, but I'm pretty sure that wouldn't be the one. How humiliating– especially if people were listening to that conversation. But it did make me laugh.

On a more exciting note, I received confirmation today that I have been selected to attend the Young Adult Conference at Camp-Mak-A-Dream in Montana. It is an all-expenses-paid trip to Gold Creek, Montana (about an hour away from Missoula) with the exception of airfare, but I'm pretty sure I can handle that. There will be forty cancer survivors attending the camp from June 18th – June 25th. We'll all be between the ages of 18 and 40 and are less than a year out from active treatment. We will participate in recreational activities and educational programming, and we have time each night to talk about cancer. I have always wanted to go to Montana, and when I heard about this, I immediately submitted an application. I think it will be cleansing for my mind, body, and soul! YAY!!!

Friday, April 17, 2009
Losing My Hair

Over the past few months, I have been experiencing more hair loss than average. I've tried to ignore it in hopes that if I don't acknowledge it, it will go away, or it won't be real. I'd like to say that this is only in my head, (and no pun intended, certainly not in the mood) but it's not. When I went to see my hairstylist last week, she made a comment about how thin my hair is in comparison to when she last saw me in January. Ugh! That made it all the more real.

My hair is typically very, very thick, but I have lost a significant amount of it. I know that it isn't noticeable to anyone looking at me, but what matters is that I notice it. When I'm standing in the shower with clumps of hair in my hands that fell out while washing it, I notice it. I see it when I have to clean out all of the hair that went down into the drain every day. I notice it when my carpet is covered in hair after blow-drying and styling it. It is incredibly distressing to me, and this morning was particularly difficult, probably because I finally realize that it is true. I can't make it go away by pretending it isn't happening. I ended up in tears this morning because I am so upset over losing so much hair and I am continuing to watch it fall out day after day. Today, I couldn't get my hair to do what I need it to do, so it's not that obvious, and I was so extremely frustrated. There could be a variety of reasons why this is happening, so figuring it out is not likely. At least that's what the nurse told me this morning when she called me about my endoscopy. It could be because of all of the anesthesia I have been given, it could be the stress, it could be the Tamoxifen, or it could be something else. Whatever the reason for it, I don't like it at all. Losing my hair to chemotherapy would have been one thing, but not knowing why I'm losing it and losing it in the amount and rate at which I'm losing it does not sit very well with me. I honestly think that I have lost enough of me over the past two years that it is time to stop. Seriously. I am not handling this well emotionally, and it most certainly didn't help matters when someone (not knowing that I've lost some of my hair but knowing enough to know better not to say what he did) asked me if we can shave my head bald before I go on the cancer retreat to Montana. *insert colorful word here*

I took a half-day off work today because I'm upset to the point of being sick to my stomach over this. I can't stop crying, so there was no real point in being there. I need to be alone for a while...to crawl back into bed, pull the blankets over my head, cry, and wish it would all go away.

Monday, April 27, 2009
Still No Answers

I had my appointment for a colonoscopy and upper endoscopy yesterday. I had to be there at 2:30 pm but wasn't scheduled to be seen until 3:30 pm. Annette went with me since I couldn't go alone. I was taken into pre-op pretty quickly after my arrival. The pre-op nurse was great with me and didn't make me cry while inserting the IV. She actually numbed my hand with Lidocaine before putting in the IV. A little before 3:30 pm, I was wheeled into the operating room for the procedure. It was freezing in there so they had to get me a warm blanket so I would stop shivering. I was chatting with the nurses while they got everything ready. One of the male nurses asked me if I was having the procedures because I was experiencing symptoms. I simply said yes and left it at that. However, another nurse blurted out, "I thought you had rectal bleeding." I know my face turned beet red and said, "Ya know, I'd rather not blurt that out for the world to know." They assured me that they wouldn't advertise it on a billboard, but it still isn't something I prefer to broadcast.

Dr. Abo came in a short time later and introduced himself again. After realizing I had seen him a little more than a month ago, he asked me why we were doing the endoscopy, so I had to explain everything again. As they were preparing me for the procedure, the nurse asked me my name one more time, and I told her I am Sally. She giggled but then told me not to joke too much because they will cancel the appointment. Okay...I'm done kidding! They gave me the oxygen and then placed a piece of hard plastic in my mouth to protect my teeth. As the anesthetist started pushing the anesthesia through my IV, I yelled because of the pain but then was out a short time after. I remember waking up in the recovery room and was rambling on about something. I was asking the names of everyone around me for some reason, and when the anesthesia nurse told me his name was Ed and not Adam, I made him give me his name tag so that I could check, although I couldn't actually see it because I was still so out of it.

I was in the recovery room for about a half-hour, I think. I saw Dr. Abo walk by as I was coming to and asked him if he found anything. He said we could chat after I wake up some more, but then he told the lady next to me that everything looked fine on hers. As I was getting ready to move to the step-down recovery room, my plastic surgeon came through the room. He did a double-take but kept walking until I said hello to him. He was trying to have a conversation with me, but it wasn't going very well because I was so doped up. He thought I might have been in surgery to have my ovaries removed, but I told him that I was not giving up my ovaries. He did ask me how things were going with the reconstruction. I told him that I'm ignoring the dropping of the right side because I don't want to go back to see him yet. I'm such an ego-booster.

I went into step-down recovery, curled up in the chair, and tried to go back to sleep. The nurse brought me some ginger ale and crackers. Annette came in to be with me. Dr. Abo stopped in to tell me he hadn't seen anything. He wants to talk to Dr. Puhalla about it to see what she would like to do. My thoughts...NO MORE TESTS!!!! Annette helped me to get dressed. The nurse indicated that I was free to go. I was taken aback that she expected me to walk to the car and said something to her about it not being a good idea for me to do that. She seemed annoyed with me, but I don't care. It was a bad idea for me to walk that distance. All I wanted was to go back to sleep. Annette met me outside and brought me home. She stayed with me for a few hours. I was fighting sleep as I was trying to watch the videos from the Emerald Dream Ball in Las Vegas, but I lost that battle and ended up passing out. She left around 7:30 pm and then Boy came over at about 9:00 pm to be with me. I had a horrible headache and woke up this morning feeling like I have a hangover. I haven't tried eating yet because my stomach is still a bit weak and I want to go back to sleep, which is where I'm going now.

Monday, May 25, 2009
Finding My Spark Again

It's been almost a month since my last journal entry...not because I don't have anything to write about, but simply because I'm ready to move beyond the all-consuming cancer journey that I've been on for the past two years. I went to see my surgical oncologist, Dr. Ahrendt, for my two-year follow up on May 5th. I had a great conversation with her about life, my health, and cancer. At one point in our conversation, she looked at me with the sincerest eyes, the most heartbroken face, and in a cracking voice said, "Melissa, you have truly been robbed." I didn't cry, even though I really wanted to because I honestly feel that way every single day. What she said went straight through me and shook the core of my being like very few things in my life have. It brought out something in me that I thought had been lost– the burning desire to make up for time lost due to all that I've been through in the past two years.

It is exciting when that part of you comes to light in this type of situation. From that day, I decided I was making it my mission to make up for the past two years of my life that has been consumed by all this cancer bullshit. I'm ready to find my own happiness– to see that rainbow and to not let cancer have such a tight grip on me anymore. I've been getting out there and taking life by the horns.

I started a book that I write at least three things I'm grateful for daily. Sometimes they are simple things. Sometimes they are much more profound, but it has been helpful for me in finding my own happiness. I have started my own "bucket list" of things I want to do before I die and keep adding to it almost every day. I take every opportunity to experience something or someone new and have been enjoying that. After two years, I've finally realized that there is still a spark in me that I thought had died when cancer came, and I'm not going to let cancer put out that spark again!

I went to the Race for the Cure on Mother's Day. It was very different for me this year because it was the first time that I was actually able to walk through it on my own two feet and coherent enough to know what was going on around me. Sadly, I liked it much better the other way. There were too many people there for my liking, and within the first fifteen minutes, some lady put her hand on the scar on my back. I wanted to jump right out of my skin. I honestly think that if you are in a crowd of breast cancer survivors, you should know better than to touch. I've accomplished my goal of not doing the race in a wheelchair three years in a row. Next year I will be having a slumber party- we will be sleeping in for the cure instead.

The hair loss has continued but has slowed down some since I started taking a supplement. Dr. Puhalla called last week and wants me to have my thyroid checked so once I feel like getting around to it, I will have the blood test done for that. I honestly don't think that is the issue, but I will entertain her thought. Nothing more is being done about the GI symptoms, so I suppose that one also gets chalked up as another "unknown" for me as well. I'd much rather have an answer than no answer, especially since I'm still having symptoms.

I have been actively involved in Today's Faces of Gilda's Club. I have two events scheduled so far. The spread on the Faces will be out in next month's Pittsburgh Magazine. I feel cheated of my own quote, though, because they gave credit to an unknown author. I used my quote from the calendar I had been a part of for Pink Profile: "Sometimes you have to walk through the rain to be able to see the rainbow." Hopefully, the commercial will be up on YouTube soon. I have raised a little more than five hundred dollars so far and hope to surpass my goal of two-thousand dollars with my first event.

My personal life has been hopping these days. It is exciting. I never thought I would be back in the dating scene or even necessarily want to be back in it for that matter. I thought Boy and I had been at a good place for some time, but recently, he has become somewhat possessive and jealous. He has frequently referred to me as his girlfriend. I have been honest with Boy from the beginning that I'm not looking for a boyfriend right now; however, Boy was hoping I would change my mind as time passed. He doesn't know me very well. He is a great guy and super sweet, but there is definitely a difference in where we are in our lives, and that tends to get in the way frequently. I think he sees a beautiful girl who is broken, and he is the right guy to fix it. He most certainly gets credit for helping me realize that I can still be beautiful and lovable despite all that I have been through, but he isn't what I would want in a long-term relationship. I feel horrible because I know I've hurt him, and that was never my intention. I can't keep going on with something that has no future when I know he is hoping for that. He recently started questioning me about some of my guy friends that I've been hanging out with, and that didn't sit well with me at all. I am not ready to be considerate of someone else's feelings in that way. My other issue is that our conversations are always superficial, and I think this has to do with the difference in our ages. I am not ever intellectually engaged in conversation with him, and I need that.

So...I met a guy (closer to my age) a few weeks ago through a mutual friend, and we have hung out about eight times in the past two weeks! I never even saw this coming. He was very standoffish with me when we first met, but then he became intrigued and fascinated by me. We could not stop talking to one another. We have great conversations, and our wittiness and humor are right in line with each other. I wasn't expecting him to like me as much as he apparently did and was caught off guard when he asked me out on a date after we had already hung out five times. We have now been on three dates...today will be the fourth. I like that he tells me how he enjoys hearing my voice and that I'm intellectually appealing to him. He actually listens to what I say, and we have yet to have a conversation that doesn't last for more than an hour. I was up until 4:00 am talking with him last night. He definitely gets bonus points for coming through on my rule of no movies and no dinner for our dates. He took me to Fun Fest, where I kicked his ass in almost every game we played. He took me to two premier parties for some of his clients, and then we went and hung out by the waterfall at the North Shore. We are going to Kennywood this evening. He gets double bonus points for actually going to two picnics with me this weekend where he knew absolutely no one but seemed to enjoy himself and be happy to be there. We definitely have a lot of fun together, and I'm always looking to increase my fun intake. I'm still not looking for a boyfriend right now, and I most certainly am not thinking about where this may go. I'm taking this for what it is worth and enjoying the time that we share together.

Happiness and laughter are my new addictions.

Tuesday, June 2, 2009
Saying Goodbye

The call came early last week that my Uncle John's health had taken a significant turn for the worse. His body was becoming brittle and frail, and the cancer was sucking the life out of him. He hadn't eaten for days on end. The decision was made to call hospice in, so I knew his fate. Without knowing how much time was left, my parents and I made the trip to Michigan on Friday to be with him before he passed. There is something creepy and unsettling about packing for a funeral for someone who has not yet passed. We arrived at about 7:00 pm on Friday night. My mom immediately went in to be with Uncle John, but I couldn't, for fear of what I might see. I stood in the kitchen sifting through pictures of him until I couldn't any longer. Then I went outside.

My Uncle Adam came out and held me in his arms as I cried. He took me by the hand and led me back to the bedroom where my Uncle John was resting. I've seen people dying from cancer before, but I was completely unprepared to see what this disease had done to my Uncle John. It hit me like never before. His body was so thin and frail, and he was not entirely coherent. I could see him trying to fight this obnoxious disease, but it had completely taken over. He could no longer walk, talk, or eat. He was slowly becoming lifeless. When given some time alone with him, I knelt down on the floor next to him, held onto his hand, and prayed to God to let him stay. I begged and pleaded with Him again that I would go instead. As I sat there, Loren and Robert ran into the room to see me, and it was like a thousand knives cutting into my heart. They knew something was wrong but didn't fully understand what it meant that their daddy was dying. My parents and I stayed for a few hours and then went to stay the night in a nearby hotel.

My mom pounded on my door early Saturday morning, telling me we had to go to my Uncle John's because his breath had become very shallow. I wasn't ready for this. My dad picked me up at the hotel, and we arrived right behind the pastor. We all gathered around my Uncle John and prayed. I cried. I showed him the shirt I wore for him that says, "Cancer Can Kiss My Ass" and though he couldn't respond, I have no doubt he appreciated it. I left the bedroom to sit in the living room in the recliner where my Uncle John often sat, pulled myself into my shell, and listened to my cancer comfort songs for most of the morning and into the afternoon. I cried so hard as Somewhere Over the Rainbow played in my ears. I went back to the bedroom to say something to my Uncle Adam and a friend of Lynette, my Uncle John's wife, asked me who I was. Before I could answer, a lady that I'd been having a hard time dealing with chimed in to say that I was Kathy's daughter and "she is John's sister but not his real sister" (because he and my mom are half-siblings). I became outraged and told her she needed to stop with the whole "real" bullshit because it wasn't the time or the place for it. It pissed me off so much that my dad had to take me away from the house before I put my hands around her throat. I know my Uncle John heard what she had said and there is no doubt in my mind that if he could have verbalized it, he would have told her that my mom is his sister and that I am his niece. He too would have been angry over that statement.

My dad and I returned to the house a little while later, when I was somewhat calmer. Pretty much the whole family was there at this point. As I was brushing my teeth and trying to use the bathroom, my mom kept banging on the door for me to come out because Lynette, my Uncle John's wife, wanted me; I had no idea why the urgency. I went into the room and was told that he had passed. I wanted to scream "God, why?" but instead held Lynette and sobbed like a baby. After several minutes, everyone left the room. It was just me with my lifeless Uncle John. I couldn't bring myself to leave his side, so I lay there next to him crying so hard that I shook the bed with every breath. I told him that I didn't want him to go, that I wanted so badly to give my life to save his, and that I loved him so much.

Several people had come in to tell me it would be okay, but they don't get it. I don't expect them to understand. I can't even begin to explain how different this has hit me and how close to home it touches me since my own diagnosis. It makes it very hard for me to understand why him and not me? Lynette came back into the room after a little while. We sat on the bed listening to Somewhere Over the Rainbow and held one another. She smiled when I said he would be sitting on the moon, watching over all of us. My parents and I never got to make it back home. We are still here and will be until the funeral on Wednesday. The days have been long and the nights even longer. I've woken up every morning with tears running down my face. I can't believe that my Uncle John is gone, and it breaks my heart every time I see his children. They are all now his life, and his legacy will be carried on through them. I will forever hold them close to my heart because that is where my Uncle John will always be.

Monday, July 6, 2009
Camp Mak-A-Dream

I haven't written in my journal for more than a month now, so I'm well overdue on an update with things. I guess it isn't a bad thing that I am not journaling as often.

I had my first "Today's Faces of Gilda's Club" event on June 13th. All things considered, it went well, and we had a blast. I am only three hundred dollars short of my goal. Funny that I accepted this challenge at the very last minute (due to concerns with having enough free time to pull off any events) and have surprised even myself with how I've taken the ball and run with it.

I went to Camp-Mak-A-Dream in Gold Creek, Montana from June 18th to the 25th. I initially had some reservations considering that I was the oldest camper and was frequently mistaken as a counselor rather than a camper, but I quickly came to appreciate my being there...not only for all the good that came out of it for me, but also for some of the relationships that I had developed in my time there. There were several activities scheduled for us throughout the day. I enjoyed the educational programs, but I particularly enjoyed those activities that took me out of my comfort zone and made me face some of my biggest fears. For starters, I am not a huge fan of horses– at all. They are massive beasts that scare the hell out of me, but I was able to get out in the field with them and lead one around. Though I had intended to ride a horse, something I've never done before on my own, I never got to because of a migraine that had me in bed for about fifteen hours.

I did the climbing wall and the high ropes course, and I hiked the mountain where the camp is nestled. I got to watch the sunset from atop the mountain one evening, which was absolutely breathtaking and tranquil. I also wore a bathing suit for the first time in more than a year. I have been so self-conscious of my scars that I couldn't bring myself to go out in public in my bikini, but toward the end of the week, I finally did. One of the most profound things that occurred while I was away at camp was that I actually started to see a side of me that everyone can see but I never could. It took meeting several people who knew very little of me for me to see and believe that there is something truly unique and special in me. There was something that I brought to the camp that no other camper had. I'm not sure exactly what it was, but it was apparent to many people and for the first time, myself. I had some great and in-depth conversations with a few of the other campers as well as some of the counselors that were eye-opening for me. It's funny how different I feel about myself after having gone there. It was probably one of the most defining moments (week, really) of my learning to accept myself for who I am and what I have

242

been through. It was great to feel like I could put everything behind me for a week. Even if it was only for a week.

While away at camp, one of my BFFs (Cathie) sent me a care package with a bunch of toys and candy. I think I'm the only camper who actually got mail. I also got a CD from Bud, the guy that I've been seeing since May. I'm not even sure what to say about it other than he truly amazes me in all that he does. I've never met anyone quite like him. He included all of the songs that remind him of me, but they told a story from our first having met right up to the point of me returning home. I sat listening to it alone and was in complete awe that someone like him has actually come into my life and wants to be a part of it- all parts of it. I missed him while I was away and made sure that I got to talk to him almost every night while I was there. Since I've returned home, we have spent a significant amount of time with one another and have yet to want to strangle each other. We spent four days together last weekend and four days together this past weekend. He has already met my parents, and I met his parents last week. I never saw this coming at all! I was pretty content with doing my thing and not letting anyone get close to me in any way, especially a guy (considering my experience with Justin). But with him, it all seems to be natural and right. It scares the hell out of me, but for some reason, I'm so much more open with him than I am with most people. I have frequently had conversations with him that have started with "I don't really know why I'm telling you this, but..."

We have great conversations, whether they are in-depth or everyday conversations, and we genuinely enjoy being in each other's company. I've always felt as though something was missing in my life and I whole-heartedly believe it has been him. I have no reservations with him. Though I don't know where this will go, I'm actually ready and willing to put myself in a place to find out.

I see my gynecological oncologist on July 10th for my six-month check-up. I will be planning to have a conversation with her about not going to Magee for any type of tests, as it is too emotionally traumatizing for me. I hope that on some level she can understand that, and we can come up with an alternate plan.

I will be going to Texas on July 23rd to the 26th to do a photoshoot for a 2010 calendar. I will be there with my friend, Crystal, whom I met in Las Vegas at the Emerald Dream Ball. She is also a model for the calendar. We are planning a few days around the shoot to hang out and for her to show me around Houston. I'm super excited!

Wednesday, July 8, 2009
Low Platelet Levels

I went to see my primary care physician, Dr. Andrews, on June 11th, as I have been experiencing a significant amount of bruising without knowing how I am getting the bruises. When I was away in Michigan, the whole left side of my leg looked like someone had beaten me, but I didn't know where any of the bruises came from. Since the radiation, I have bruised much more easily, worse, and more deeply than I had in the past. I can still see residual bruises on my legs from when I was going through radiation. I figured that since I'm almost two years out from the radiation, I should probably see Dr. Andrews to explore what might be causing my bruising. He recommended I have blood work done to check my blood count and platelets, which I completed on June 12th. I hadn't heard anything from him since then, so I called yesterday to see if there were any results as of yet. I would like to think that no news is good news, but I never take my chances with that these days. Dr. Andrews hadn't yet received the results, probably because I had two scripts for blood work when I went down to Magee. Once Dr. Andrew's office was able to call Magee to get the results, Dr. Andrews called me back to let me know that my blood count is good, but my platelet levels are below average. He wants me to have another blood test done to determine if my platelet levels are progressively dropping or to see if they are back at normal levels. Several things can cause my platelet levels to be low, so if they continue to be below the average range or are showing a progressive drop, he will refer me to a hematologist for further evaluation.

Friday, July 10, 2009
Ovarian Cysts, Uterine Lining Concerns, and Endometrial Cancer

I went to see Dr. Zorn, my gynecological oncologist, today. I'd been kind of stepping out of the cancer world a little bit and pretending as though it doesn't exist. I don't want it to become the issue that forces its way between Bud and me, so I've been ignoring it. Today, the reality that it still exists and continues to be an issue I need to deal with slapped me in the face, again. I'd been on such a natural high with everything in my life over the past two months that I kind of came crashing down after my visit with Dr. Zorn.

I only did the ultrasound today and will do the CA-125 when I go back in January. My CA-125 last time was 29. The level at which they would start to become concerned is 31...not good. Today was the first time in all of my appointments that I actually felt like Dr. Zorn cared about what I had to say. She said that there is a cyst on my left ovary that she feels may be related to ovulating, so we will monitor that. Dr. Zorn is more concerned with my uterine lining, which led into a lengthy discussion about the one topic I hate the most, the removal of my ovaries. She wanted to know how I felt about having my ovaries out, and I adamantly indicated I have no intentions of removing them prophylactically, ever. Since I have no plans of removing my ovaries, Dr. Zorn noted that we need to continue monitoring the uterine lining and if necessary, conduct a biopsy. If the biopsy reveals that it is hyperplasia (which is a pre-cancer) or that there is endometrial cancer, she will recommend that I have a hysterectomy and removal of my ovaries and my fallopian tubes.

I sat there in a daze for a moment taking it all in. So, I would lose my uterus, my ovaries, and my fallopian tubes. Seriously? Can't I get a fucking break on this cancer bullshit? It seems as though my body continues to be my own worst enemy. Eventually, I will be forced to have everything removed whether I want to or not. I get the whole thing about getting rid of cancer and not allowing it to take over my body, but at the same time, there is a part of me that wants to be shallow and vain and keep the remaining female body parts that I have. There are times when I don't feel worthy of being called a woman, and I don't expect anyone to understand that...unless you have been through what I have been through. I'm so angry and frustrated over the fact that I keep looking for an end and there has yet to be one.

I brought it to Dr. Zorn's attention that I cannot emotionally handle going to Magee for the ultrasounds because of all of the pregnant women that are there. I look at them and so wish that I could be one of them. I want to be sitting there with the person I love so dearly holding me, wearing big, glowing smiles on our faces as we wait to see our baby and listen to its heartbeat. I started to cry, and for the first time, she heard me say, "But, that will never be me." This, of course, led into the baby conversation. I became somewhat frustrated with her because I have done a significant amount of research on this and have thought long and hard about my decision. It's certainly not the decision that I wanted to be forced into making, but it is what I feel is right for me. I explained to her that I've considered all options and having a baby without any type of intervention would be selfish on my part, despite what everyone thinks may occur in the future regarding the advances in medicine.

My retort to that is my Great-Grandmother had a bilateral mastectomy, and so did I; medicine hasn't advanced that much. I'm not willing to take that chance. Honestly, I could never bear the guilt of seeing my child go through what I have been through. It certainly would be a recipe for my own disaster. There is the option of storing my eggs and evaluating them to see if they carry the gene and then destroying those that have the gene and preserving those that do not but they would have to increase the levels of estrogen in my body, which is counterproductive to the Tamoxifen and puts me at risk for developing more cancer. There is also the option of adopting, but there are also challenges that can come along with that as well. I don't think either of them is an option for me right now.

This all then got me thinking about Bud and how I can see us being together down the road...I don't know how far down the road but still, I see it. I am sad for him that should it go that far, having children will never be a part of his reality, either. We actually had this conversation because I figured that it would be easier for him to get out now if having children is something he has his heart set on. I was taken aback when he told me that he always imagined himself with children and that he had thought very long and hard about how much that meant to him since I'd made several comments in general conversation about not having kids. Bud said that he thought about whether the person he would be with was worth him not having children, and he decided that I am. But there is still a level of guilt that I feel because I know it is something he had wanted in his life. I not only feel sad for him but for me, as well. I can only say again that life truly isn't fair for reasons that I cannot understand. They say that God never promises life to be fair; He promises it will be worth it. I hope that it is!

Saturday, August 1, 2009
Pink Door Calendar Photo Shoot

At the end of July, I went to Texas to do another calendar shoot. It was for the Pink Door Foundation. The calendar will be revealed in October 2009.

My friend, Crystal, and I spent Friday doing some damage to the pocketbooks! We shopped almost all day and had a wonderful time. On Saturday, we had the photoshoot. It is a pretty cool idea that they came up with for the calendar. It is black and white, but the painting they put on my shoulder of the half pink ribbon, half teal ribbon in the shape of a heart will be in color. I got to work with a male model that apparently ended up having a crush on me. Funny!

After the shoot, Crystal and I had lunch with another model in the calendar. That night, we went to the Kemah Boardwalk to have dinner with Crystal's friend. We stopped by NASA space center along the way, and I was in my glory even though I didn't get to go inside. I've always been interested in space and science, so it was exciting to be standing outside of the facility. We had a great time at dinner and walking on the boardwalk.

Crystal and I had a talk that evening about something very near and dear to my heart– leaving behind a legacy. She has a daughter, and her legacy will always live on in her, but I've accepted the responsibility of carrying on her mission related to breast cancer in black women. Crystal had vowed to me that should I pass before her, she will carry on my legacy and my passion for increasing awareness of cancer in young women, early screening/detection, and adequate healthcare. It meant so much to me that she would accept that responsibility because I frequently think about what my legacy would be if that day came sooner than later that I'm no longer a part of the Earthly world. When I left on Sunday, we promised that we would make an attempt to see one another once a year and try to get some of the other Emerald Dream Ball girls to join us.

Monday, August 17, 2009
Blood Work and Painful Foobies

On August 6th, I went for additional blood work to test my platelet levels again to see if I need to see a hematologist, but I haven't gotten the results back yet. I called this week, but Dr. Andrews hadn't received anything. I will call again next week.

I also went to see my plastic surgeon, Dr. Gimbel, that day because I've been experiencing significant pain in my chest, and the right side is lower than the left. He didn't seem too concerned with the right side being as low as it is...I'm the only one that doesn't like it. His concern is that I look symmetrical in clothing...not out of them. Easy enough for him to say.

He asked me about how the reconstruction looked in a bathing suit and seemed shocked when I told him I've only been in a bathing suit once since my last surgery. I was so self-conscious about being in it that I didn't even think about how symmetrical I looked. I think that might have finally been the thing that made him realize how hard this has all been for me. I explained that I totally avoid situations where I might need to wear a bathing suit because of all the scars.

As for the pain, he indicated that it's likely the result of the radiation. Though I was told that the effects of the radiation would only last for a year after my last treatment, what he said made much more sense to me. The radiation damaged the tissue in the area that was irradiated. Thus, it can never fully heal or recover. He told me that the pain will likely get worse as the years continue on, it will never get better. Well, that's fun and exciting. I'm probably going to be a pain killer junky in a few years. He did say that he is pleased with the how the scar from my latissimus surgery looks and he seems to think that things look pretty good (everyone is entitled to their own perception and opinion, I suppose). I will see him again in a year.

I have my next appointment in September with my medical oncologist for a check-up.

Friday, August 21, 2009
Relationship Status: Taken

I'm hosting another event for Today's Faces of Gilda's Club next Thursday at the Hard Rock Cafe. It is a belly dance performance and a jewelry fashion show. I'm excited about the event and am hoping to have a full house. The day after, Bud and I leave for the weekend to go to North Carolina. I'm meeting his brother and sister-in-law, and we are going to stay at his uncle's beach house in Myrtle Beach.

I suppose that for the first time since 2006, I would say I'm in a relationship. It still makes me nervous, but I'm trying hard not to let my fear of the unknown impact how I live for today. I frequently ask Bud about the "what ifs" and he is adamant that he will always be here. What breaks my heart, though is that when I think about the "what ifs," I know he would be completely devastated without me. My parents seem to like him, though they haven't had much time to get to know him. It's a pretty big deal if my dad thinks he is a nice guy. He treats me like no other guy I've ever been in a relationship with...he is thoughtful, considerate, respectful, and head over heels for me. He talks openly with me about everything and wants to know all of the ins and outs of Melissa. I think I shall keep him around.

A song recently released by Kenny Chesney and Dave Matthews, "I'm Alive", touches me deeply and reminds me to live for today, every day.

"So damn easy to say that life's so hard. Everybody's got their fair share of battle scars. As for me, I'd like to thank my lucky stars that I'm alive and well.

It'd be easy to add up all the pain and all the dreams you sat and watched go up in flames. Dwell on the wreckage as it smolders in the rain. But not me, I'm alive.

And today, you know that's good enough for me. Breathing in and out is a blessing can't you see. Today's the first day of the rest of my life. I'm alive and well. Yeah, I'm alive and well.

Stars are dancing on the water here tonight. It's good for the soul when there's not a soul in sight. This boat has caught its wind and brought me back to life. Now I'm alive and well.

And today you know that's good enough for me. Breathing in and out is a blessing, can't you see. Today is the first day of the rest of my life. Now I'm alive and well. Yeah I'm alive and well."

Such a short and simple song but so profound!

Saturday, September 1, 2009
Belly Dancing and In-Laws

My "Legends and Inspirations" show at the Hard Rock Cafe went well, and I raised almost fourteen hundred dollars! I was nervous but did well, I suppose. I was excited to have my family and friends there to support me. My friend Rick Hill, whom I met in Montana at Camp-Mak-A-Dream, drove all the way from Minnesota to be there for my show. I was so very touched that he thought that much of me and drove all that way.

Things went okay with meeting Bud's brother. I was a big ball of stress. I felt like there were such high expectations that I was always on edge. I had several moments where I became the sassy-ass Melissa that people either love or hate, so it wasn't all fun times. His brother and sister-in-law are very cool. We definitely have different interests than they do, but it was still fun. For all the hype that surrounds Myrtle Beach, I can honestly say I wasn't all that impressed with it.

Thursday, September 10, 2009
Medical Oncology Appointment

I went to see Dr. Puhalla, my medical oncologist. My appointment took two hours for no good reason at all. I would have been content with sitting there reading my Gilda Radner book It's Always Something, but I was freezing even with the heated blanket from the chemo room. The nurse practitioner came in to see me first. We chatted for a bit about some random things and then discussed the pain I continue to have in my back, my back door, my pelvic area, and now my chest. She was concerned and thought that Dr. Puhalla may order more tests, but I told her that I'm not interested in going through any more testing only to have it show up as nothing. I know it is there, and I will simply deal with the pain. I waited for what seemed like forever for Dr. Puhalla to get there. I tried to hold having to go to the bathroom until I finished with my appointment, but I couldn't wait any longer. I had to go out in the hallway in my robe (extra-large and open in the front) to find a bathroom...I swear my back teeth were floating.

Finally, Dr. Puhalla showed up and apologized for the length of time I waited for her. We talked about the clinical trial that she is conducting to prevent breast cancer and ovarian cancer cells from dividing. I do not qualify for the trial because it is only for Stage IV (metastatic) cancers. Of course, I was happy that I didn't qualify but sad that it isn't available to help prevent additional breast cancer or the development of ovarian cancer in patients like me. She thinks it will impact future generations. We talked about the pain as well. I told her that I don't want to go through any more testing to find that nothing shows up on any of the tests. I explained that I have come to the terms that I will likely become a pain pill junkie in the future. She offered me a prescription for pain medication, but I declined because I still refuse to take anything. I have to be in some severe pain to take even over-the-counter meds. She indicated that my sensation in and around my chest may be changing, which could be causing some of the pain. Plus, I continue to have issues related to the lasting effects of radiation. She examined me and indicated that everything looked good. I will see her again in three months.

I see the radiation oncologist, Dr. Beriwal, in November for my two-year check-up.

Monday, September 14, 2009
Exciting News

I finally got the results from my blood work. My platelets continue to be low but have shown some improvement since June. Dr. Andrews would like for me to go back to get them checked in again in three months.

On a more exciting note, I am working with a local designer to create a t-shirt I'm hoping to launch in October for breast cancer awareness month. I have seen the design and must say it is pretty cool. I mean, it will have my name on it so how much cooler can it really get? A portion of the proceeds will be donated to a breast cancer charity of my choice with the hope that eventually some of those proceeds will go toward the non-profit organization that I'm trying to get up and running. It's all still in the works, but I do believe it will eventually come to fruition.

Tuesday, November 10, 2009
Thank You, Cancer?

Wow! It has been almost two months since I have written in my journal.

I had an appointment with my radiation oncologist, Dr. Beriwal, on November 2nd. He wasn't in the office that day, so I had to see another doctor, which is frustrating because I end up having to tell my story all over again. I was seen by the Physician's Assistant first. After the Twenty Questions game with her, Diane, my favorite nurse in the office, came in to see me. She always makes me feel so good when I'm there. We talked briefly about what and how I'm doing these days. The doctor came in shortly after Diane and performed the regular exam that my radiation oncologist performs. Diane stood next to me and held my hand the whole time. It reminded me that even though I've come this far in my journey and I can finally see the light at the end of the tunnel, I still am very much frightened by the thought of one of my doctors finding something again. It was nice to have someone comfort those fears that I work so hard to suppress day in and day out. The doctor indicated that everything looked fine and said that the reconstruction was well done. When asked about my feelings regarding the reconstruction, I responded with my usual, "I'd much rather have my own."

I have learned to accept what has happened to me, but that does not ever mean that I have to like it. Both seemed to acknowledge that my feelings over the reconstruction were justified. The doctor finished up the exam and indicated that I would need to return in another year. Two years down, three more years of check-ups with the radiation oncologist to go! Woo Hoo!!

Since I was already at Magee, I decided to get my blood work done to check on my platelet levels. I'm hoping they come back better than before, but I'm not too hopeful because I have been bruising a lot lately. I suppose I will have to wait and see.

I will see my gynecological oncologist, Dr. Zorn, in January. I'm not looking forward to that appointment at all. Given all the issues I've had with my who-ha, I have a feeling that there will be a lot of pressure for me to have my ovaries removed, along with the fallopian tubes and possibly my uterus. I still have not changed my mind. I'm still not ready, and I don't see that changing over the next seven months– when I turn 35.

A few things are going on that I'm pretty excited about these days. On November 21st, I will be sharing my story at the Curves in Burgettstown. They are hosting a benefit for the American Cancer Society and asked me to be the speaker. On December 3rd, I will be speaking at a medical conference on the BRCA1/2 mutation in Pittsburgh, and on December 8th, I will be sharing my story with the Pitt medical students.

In addition to that, I am currently in the infantile stage of starting an organization called Cancer Fighting Princess. We launched a Facebook fan page in October. At this point, we have more than three thousand fans on our Facebook fan page. My very dear and talented friend, Amanda, donated her time to help design our logo (which is very cute and very Melissa-like). Bud has been the mastermind behind everything, and we have had a great response to it thus far.

Speaking of Bud *deep breath in, deep breath out*, things are going exceptionally well with us. We have pretty much spent every single day together since June after my return from Montana. He picked me up from the airport that night, brought me home, and never left. Since we pretty much live together already, we decided to get a place together. So as of December 1st, *deep breath in, deep breath out*, we will be living together in a house in Allison Park. I must admit I'm nervous because I have never moved in with someone. I have lived with someone that I had dated for a very long time, but he moved into my place with me, and we had our own bedrooms (should have been the red flag that that relationship wasn't going to last). Bud and I have talked about marriage, and I do believe that one day that will happen, sometime in the near, distant future.

Finally! I have found that somebody who loves me for me, despite all that I have been through and without any level of doubt, will be here for me should I have to face this journey again. I feel as though my life is finally starting (or my second life, anyway). Though things will never be what they were, I am beginning to find my "new" normal because of him. Though I think about cancer every day, it certainly is no longer the first thing I think of in the morning nor the last thing I think of when I go to bed at night. I'm still terrified of cancer coming back. I have had dreams that I'm in the last stages of my life, begging not to go and telling Bud that I don't want to leave him. I will take every single day with him for what it is worth. I will love him and appreciate our time together, no matter how short or long that may be. I have said all along that everything happens for a reason and I whole-heartedly believe that because if I had never had cancer, I probably would have never met him. I never thought I would say this but THANK YOU, CANCER!!

Saturday, December 19, 2010
Sharing My Story

Toward the end of November, I spoke at a cancer benefit hosted by the Curves in Burgettstown, PA. It was probably my most challenging speech as my mother and Aunt Aggie were sitting right in the front row with tears streaming down their faces as I shared my story and displayed pictures of my journey. However, I'd had a few shots of Sangria beforehand, so that was somewhat helpful.

At the beginning of December, I shared my story at the Heredity Cancers conference hosted by an oncologist from Shadyside Hospital. This was a very different audience for me as it consisted of doctors and residents from all walks of oncology, geneticists, etc. Even my gynecological oncologist was sitting in the audience. I was surprised when I looked into the crowd and saw many men and women with red, tear-filled eyes as I shared my story. I hadn't expected to hit a nerve with any of them. After all, they see this day in and day out, so I figured my story was nothing special to any of them. I can't tell you how many of them came up to me after and told me, "thank you." They found it helpful and very touching. Even Dr. McDreamy (that's what they call him at Shadyside...and trust me, he is dreamy) came over to say thanks. In appreciation for sharing my story, I got free Penguins tickets to the game at Mellon Arena that night. Bud and I went to the game and sat in the Club Seats, which in my opinion are the worst seats in the entire arena, as they are all the way at the top, but the game was fun, and I appreciated the opportunity to be there.

On December 8th, I spoke to the University of Pittsburgh medical students again. I find doing that so very rewarding. It was nice to hear the professor tell me that of all the things her students had experienced last year, hearing my story was one of the most memorable for them. I hope that it stays with them for a long time to come so that when they are dealing with their patients, they can show some compassion. A number of the students came to me after I was done speaking to thank me. There was one guy in particular who had caught my attention. He was sitting in the front row, asked a lot of questions, and when he came to thank me, he had tears in his eyes. I hugged him because I felt compelled to do so. Later, I found out his mom had recently been diagnosed with cancer and has been caring for her while going to school. My heart broke for him.

Sunday, January 24, 2010
The Dread Ovarian Cancer Screening

On January 8th, I went to see Dr. Zorn, my gynecological oncologist, for my biannual ovarian cancer screening. It was a standard appointment. The good news is that everything looks stable. She didn't see any worsening of the ovaries or the uterine lining, which is good, but certainly doesn't explain the pelvic pain I'm having almost daily. It feels as though Charlie is always lingering around...like he may stop in for a visit at any moment. Dr. Zorn reminded me that I have six months until I turn 35. She strongly recommended that I reconsider having my ovaries removed. They must not know me very well. I've made my decision, and I'm not budging from it. I feel like the clock is ticking and the pressure is on, but I'm still not going to change my mind.

She talked with me about Bud and my relationship with him. I told her that he thinks (well, knows) he wants to marry me. I am the one afraid of commitment. She asked if we had discussed how we would avoid an unplanned pregnancy, as that would be devastating to me. Dr. Zorn thinks I should consider some type of birth control, but most, if not all, were hormonal so they aren't options for me...I have to admit I wasn't listening to this part. Then she said, "Maybe your boyfriend should consider getting snipped." I laughed so hard, I thought I might pee my pants. I certainly would never ask him to do that for me. I mean, it's my body that is trying to kill me, not his, so I don't see why he would go through such a thing. I told her I would let him know about it, though. I ended up having to get my blood taken twice, so both arms got a beating that day. I had 6 vials of blood taken for the CA-125 and the clinical trial, and then another one to check my platelets. My CA-125 came back slightly lower than last time, which is good. My platelets are below average again, which is a bummer because I had dental surgery scheduled, but they canceled it. I have to go back in March to have my platelets rechecked.

This month, I was featured in an article in Total Body Magazine out of Houston, Texas, for my involvement with the Pink Door Foundation.

I have another calendar out, but it's not anything specific to cancer. It is for the Wedding Dress Project with photographer Tom Darby.

Cancer Fighting Princess is coming along. We have a strong fan base on Facebook with more than four thousand fans. At the end of the month, we will be selling t-shirts, and I will be doing a photoshoot with the designer of the shirts.

Sunday, June 6, 2010
The Rollercoaster of Life

The past five months have had some ups and downs. I have had positive appointments with my oncologists, and there are no concerns in that regard. I fell into somewhat of a depression during January, February, and March. I pretty much isolated myself from everything. I would get up, go to work, come home, and go to sleep. It was awful for me and for Bud, who knew that something was wrong, but couldn't figure out what it was. Things started to get a little better in April. I bought a townhouse at the beginning of April, and we moved in at the end of the month. I love the new place, and it has helped to pull me out of the depression.

In early May, I went to see a gynecological specialist, Dr. Suketu Mansuria. This was at the recommendation of my regular gynecologist who seemed to think that my doctors have been so concerned with the possibility of ovarian cancer that they may have been overlooking the possibility of endometriosis as the cause for my constant pelvic pain. When I met with the specialist, he indicated that there are several ways to try to figure out the cause of the pain but because I'm a cancer survivor I cannot go the hormone therapy route, so my only option is laparoscopic surgery. He told me that I will have to have four incisions from this procedure. His course of action will be dependent on what he finds. He understands that he is only permitted to remove my ovaries if, and only if, he finds cancer. If he finds endometriosis, he is only allowed to do what is necessary to remove it, but if Dr. Mansuria finds nothing, he will cut the nerves to my uterus to stop the constant pelvic pain. Of course, there are side effects that come with cutting the nerves that are less than desirable, such as the constant feeling of having to pee. Seriously, I can't win. I am scheduled for the surgery on July 13th and will be on leave from work for two weeks to recover. I have been ignoring the fact that in a month I will be undergoing another surgery, but I know that as the time gets closer, my mind is going to wander, and the frustration and anger will seep out.

I didn't participate in the Race for the Cure this year. I registered and helped to raise money for the event, but I couldn't be there. Instead, I was at PNC Park as the Honorary Bat Girl for the Pittsburgh Pirates. I shared my story on the Major League Baseball website, had all of my friends and family vote for me, and was selected! The Pirates paid for me and 14 of my family members and friends to go to the game. We were provided the opportunity to go down on the field and meet some of the staff. We also got to meet Lastings Milledge and JR, the manager. As the Honorary Bat Girl, I was given a jersey and a pink bat. I even got to deliver the lineup card to the umpire. I had a radio interview, a locker room interview, and a live interview on Fox Sports Network. It was an exciting and busy day. The Pirates sent me a ton of photos from my day as Honorary Bat Girl, a necklace, and Lastings Milledge's pink gloves. It was definitely a day to remember.

May 17th was even more of a day to remember. I suppose in some way I have been hesitant to write about this for fear that it could be too good and something terrible would soon come to follow, as seems to be my history. This day was mine and Bud's one-year anniversary of our first date. We didn't have any set plans. I decided I wasn't going to dragon boating practice that night because of the rain, so I asked him if he wanted to go to the Olive Garden. He agreed. On the way home, it started pouring rain, so I texted him and asked him to come outside. He asked me to go inside. I told him it was raining and that I just wanted to go, so he said okay, but I could tell that he wanted me to come inside. I went in to go to the bathroom and see what he had up his sleeve. When I went into the house, he had three roses and three candles sitting on the stairs and rose petals up the steps. When I got to the second floor, there was a trail of rose petals around the love seat and into the living room where he was sitting on the other couch. He had a hundred tea lights lit around the living and dining rooms. On the coffee table sat a circle of tea lights with a pencil and note that he had written to me a year ago. The note was one of those silly things between the two of us. It was like what you did in fifth grade when you wanted to know if someone liked you. It said, "Do you like me?" with three boxes for yes, no, or maybe and was folded up into a football shape. He asked me to open it, but I thought I already knew what it said. When I opened it, he had added- "I love you, baby, with all my heart. Will you marry me?" and two boxes for yes or no. He also wrote, "immediate response required." I was in complete and utter shock and looked at him with tears in my eyes. He pulled a ring box from behind him, and I knew he wasn't kidding. I said, "Yes!"

I got engaged!! So many emotions and thoughts ran through me. I sat thinking about where I was not so long ago, thinking that no one would ever love me and that I wouldn't ever be good enough for anyone. I felt so cheated by life. We sat there hugging one another for what seemed like forever and when we released, I realized that he, too, was teary-eyed. For the past three years, I have walked through the storm; for the most part, it has been a lonely journey. But last year, I found someone who has held my hand through that storm. The storm has now passed, and the clouds have faded. Sometimes it still drizzles, but I have someone standing here holding my hand, loving me for who I am, not what I've been through.

Saturday, July 24, 2010
Endometriosis

I underwent the laparoscopic surgery on July 13th (wasn't all that excited to have it so close to my birthday) to find out what might be causing all of the pain. My surgery was scheduled for 10:00 am at Passavant Hospital, which is about fifteen minutes from our townhouse. Bud and I arrived promptly, and I was taken back to get prepped for surgery. Bud was not permitted to join me for almost forty minutes. I was ready to go for surgery at 10:00 am, but there were some complications with the case before mine, so I did not go into the operating room until almost noon. I had changed my mind about having my nerves clipped if there was no endometriosis found, which changed some things for the surgery, but nothing significant. I'm not exactly sure how long the surgery took, but it took me some time to come out of recovery, as usual. I remember the nurses trying to wake me several times without much luck. It was the same old, "Time to get up, Melissa," but I simply ignored it. The nurse that was tending to me went to lunch, and I was left at the mercy of a nurse that seemed agitated with my inability to be roused. I asked for ice chips twice before my request was honored.

Dr. Mansuria told Bud that he found a significant amount of endometriosis near my rectum. He had to place a rod in my rectum to move it to avoid causing any injury while removing the endometriosis. Dr. Mansuria also said he found a cyst on my right ovary that he removed to test for cancer given my BRCA2 status.

When I was taken to "step-down" recovery, they put me in a real room, which was nice. After about an hour and a half, I was discharged and sent along my way. I was still pretty nauseous, so I asked for a puke container to go. Bud filled my prescription for Percocet, and we went home. The Percocet didn't sit very well with me, and I threw up several times. I called in the next day for a prescription of Vicodin and was able to get one. I was off work for two weeks. During that time, I was pretty sore and moved pretty slowly, but Bud took good care of me. I was super bloated and gassy from the carbon dioxide they pumped into my stomach. So attractive, I know. I have three small incisions in my pelvic area and one in my bellybutton. After about two weeks, my bellybutton started oozing some green/yellow goop, so I went in to see Dr. Mansuria before my scheduled check-up. As luck would have it, I was allergic to the stitches, so they had to be removed.

Friday, August 20, 2010
Post-Op Follow-Up

When I went back for my one-month check-up with Dr. Mansuria, gynecological specialist, last week, he told me that I had a lot of endometriosis near my rectum. He said it was a deep pocket that likely has been growing over several years. The cyst came back benign, which was great news. I don't need to go back to see Dr. Mansuria unless there are any other concerns. I will likely have some pain, particularly during my monthly visits from Charlie, considering that he put a huge hole in my body. Indeed, he was right! Even though I've had some pain during that time, I have not had the daily, constant pelvic pain that I had experienced over the past two years. It is such a great feeling!!!

Friday, August 6, 2010
Keynote Speaker

On July 31st, I went to Shreveport, Louisiana, as the keynote speaker for the Susan G. Komen Survivor Luncheon. My friend Crystal is on the board for the Shreveport Chapter of Komen and asked if I would be willing to share my story. Without any hesitation, I accepted. They flew me down and paid for my hotel room for the night. This was probably the biggest crowd I have spoken to thus far; it was quite intimidating. The room was full of breast cancer survivors, their families, physicians, and local politicians. Before I was introduced to share my story, they surprised me with a proclamation from the mayors of Bossier City and Shreveport declaring July 31, 2010 as Cancer Fighting Princess Day. How cool is that?

There was laughter, and there were tears from men, women, and children, as I shared my story. As I was talking about my not ever having children and how much that pains me, I looked up to see my friend Crystal in tears and in the arms of a friend. She too knows the pain of not being able to have a child at the hands of cancer, as she was a newlywed when diagnosed with cancer and due to chemotherapy, she and her husband will not be able to have a child together. Even though she has an amazing daughter from a previous relationship, I know she would love to have another child with her husband. The luncheon ended with a fashion show, and I was the last to go out; I was wearing a beautiful ball gown that I wish I could have stuffed in my suitcase to bring home with me. Crystal had asked that I not talk about my recent engagement in my story, as they wanted to end the fashion show by telling everyone my good news as they played Beyoncé's Single Ladies (Put a Ring on It). I had so much fun with it as I danced around the tables and even busted out some of the moves from Beyoncé's music video. They ate it up! I got to spend another day with Crystal, and we explored Shreveport, which I didn't realize is a big area for filming movies. We went sightseeing, ate, drank, and of course did some shopping!

Saturday, October 23, 2010
Dragon Boating, NYC, and Wedding Planning

At the end of September, I went to the Mercer Park Dragon Boat Festival to compete with my Pink Steel teammates. We took first place in the breast cancer competition and came in second overall, which is incredible considering that we were competing against "healthy" women. I have my first gold medal!!

In mid-October, my best friend Chris and I went to NYC for The SCAR Project exhibit. After several years of shooting and almost a hundred women, David Jay finally had his exhibition. I was one of thirty women chosen to be displayed in the exhibit, and I'm also in the book that he has released. My BFF, Chris, and I went up early on Friday morning and stayed until late afternoon on Sunday. My cousin Joe, whom I have not seen in well over fifteen years let us stay at his place for free in Queens while he was vacationing in Mexico. Chris and I went into the city on Friday. We had lunch at the Hard Rock Cafe and had a great time. We both got a Pop Princess drink, which came with a free pilsner glass. Since neither of us drink very often, we were both tipsy...at 1:00 in the afternoon. It made for an interesting walk around the city, that is for sure. I was able to smooth talk the waitress at Hard Rock into giving me four more pilsner glasses. SCORE! As we were walking around the city, we were repeatedly stopped by guys on the street asking us if we wanted to go to a comedy show. I kept telling them that Chris didn't have a sense of humor. We did some pretty good damage shopping in the city. I think I came home with two new pairs of shoes, two scarves, and two purses. It was great.

On Saturday, we walked around Chinatown and Greenwich Village before heading over to the exhibit in the early evening. My friends, Flora and Jeffrey whom I had met in Las Vegas at the Emerald Dream Ball, came over from New Jersey to go to the exhibit with us. Before we even walked into the show, I was overflowing with emotions. It is hard to explain what it felt like to look through the window and see my picture hanging on the back wall. I had a thousand emotions running through me. It was bittersweet in so many ways. As we were doing the gallery walk, I was in tears. At one point, David Jay asked if anyone wanted to lead the gallery walk and Flora so kindly selected me. I, of course, went over to my photo. David Jay asked me to share a little bit about my story, and so I did. I was crying the whole time. It was hard to look at my photo, but at the same time, I couldn't stop. It was painful to look back into the crowd and see my friends with tear-filled eyes too. Several other girls who took part in the project that shared their story as well. At some level, it brought a sense of closure for me to that part of my life. I wasn't sure I would have ever been able to look back at that photo and not see it as something that had complete control over my life, but I was, and I was filled with a sense of relief that finally, I can move forward from that dark place.

The entire time I was there, I was texting Bud. He couldn't be there because he was at a wedding. I could tell that he would have given anything in the world to be there with me. After the gallery walk, we all went out to dinner. Chris and I did a little more shopping and then headed back to my cousins for the rest of the night. On Sunday, we explored my cousin's neighborhood and then headed to the airport to make our way back home. It was a great trip with great friends. Not only was it therapeutic for me to go, but I realized that I have some awesome friends that care about me. Chris has three little ones at home and left them for the weekend to go with me to the exhibit. I think it speaks volumes of how special our relationship is.

Onto the wedding...
Plans are coming along! We are getting married on July 16th, which is the day before my birthday and two days before Bud's birthday. We are getting married in Erie because it is WAY cheaper to get married there than anywhere in Pittsburgh. We are having a big wedding with five bridesmaids, two junior bridesmaids, and a flower girl. I have my dress; it has pink in it, of course. The girls have their dresses too; they will be in silver and pink. We have the venue, the photographer, and the DJ. I'm working on getting the officiant and the wedding cake. I also need to plan the rehearsal dinner. We registered for our wedding gifts, which was exhausting, but it is done. The big day seems so far away, but I know it will come quickly. I'm hoping that all of my hard work pays off in the end!

Monday, November 15, 2010
Just One More Thing...

After having my surgery in July to remove the endometriosis, Dr. Mansuria indicated that I would likely continue to have some pain considering the holes that he put in my body to remove all of the endometriosis. Every month since my surgery, I have had excruciating pain in my rectal area particularly when I need to have a bowel movement but only during the time of the month when Charlie visits (sorry! I hate talking about this) which is one of the symptoms that led me to having the surgery in the first place. Given that it has been four months now since my surgery, I figured I should call Dr. Mansuria and find out if this is normal. I started my period this past Saturday, and that day and into Sunday, I was having awful pain. It is enough to stop me from doing whatever I am doing at the moment. On a scale of one to ten, I would definitely put it at about an eight. That kind of pain is not normal! When I called Dr. Mansuria's office, he recommended that I have a gastrointestinal evaluation done and that I start taking fiber twice a day (I already eat a lot). I would be lying to say that I was not disappointed. I was hoping he would say to give it a few more months and call back. So here we go again!!! I have an appointment at Magee for January 3rd to meet with the digestive disorder specialist in hopes of figuring out what is going on with my bum. I know I certainly shouldn't complain, but it always seems to be one thing after another. I was hoping for one full year of not having to see any other doctors besides my usual list of docs, but apparently, that isn't going to happen. I am coming up on year four of my health going to shit (pun definitely intended). I'm so over it!

Monday, January 3, 2011
Maybe I Have a Digestive Disorder?

I met with a digestive disorder specialist because of the pain I continue to have that I had hoped would go away after having the endometriosis removed. The doctor seemed to be quite perplexed over my situation. We spent a rather long time discussing possible diagnoses, most of which made no sense because the pain typically only occurs during my periods. Initially, she suggested that I begin taking MiraLAX to soften my stool in case that is what is causing the issue and then undergo a procedure that sounded less appealing than running naked through my neighborhood. It had something to do with a balloon in my bowel while I'm awake. Hmm... After further discussion, the doctor brought up the possibility that in very few instances, the endometriosis can be found inside of the bowel. She seemed to think that though it is very rare, it is the only thing that makes sense given the cyclical nature of my pain. UGH! I learned that endometriosis can actually be found in any organ within the body. How crazy is that??

In researching endometriosis in the bowel, it turns out that a bowel resection may be necessary. WTF??? This is a pretty hefty surgery and actually is one that requires an extended hospital stay than the mastectomy or the latissimus flap procedure. The doctor suggested I contact the office as soon as possible at the beginning of my next period to get me scheduled for a scope of my bowel within the first few days. The irony is that Charlie decided to show up two weeks early this month...right in time for that appointment, but she couldn't do the scope right then. So, right now, I'm at the mercy of Mother Nature.

Friday, January 7, 2011
Six-Month Ovarian Cancer Screening

I went for my six-month check-up with Dr. Zorn, my gynecological oncologist. It was a pretty routine appointment. They asked me to have my blood drawn for the CA-125 first. The girl that works in Dr. Zorn's office is relatively young, and I was sure that she would not have gotten me on the first jab, which would have put me in a bad mood for the rest of the day. I told her that I'm usually a hard one, so after checking both arms, she decided to take me across the hall to the lab. The lady seemed somewhat irritated with both of us, but I told her that I'm not an easy stick, and she changed her attitude. They took six vials of blood!! I then went for my ultrasound, which was uneventful. The technician told me that she didn't see anything of concern but would have Dr. Zorn take a look at the films.

Dr. Zorn came in after a few minutes and reviewed everything with me. For once, there was no concern with my endometrial lining! YAY!! She said that everything looked good. I do have two cysts; one on each ovary, but she didn't have any concerns. We talked about Cancer Fighting Princess and the wedding plans. I told her I would be in to see her before the wedding in July. I left the office feeling really good about the appointment since this was the first appointment that we didn't have the discussion about having my ovaries removed and nothing came up as a concern.

Wednesday, January 12, 2011
Elevated CA-125

I got a voicemail yesterday that thought it was Dr. Puhalla's office reminding me of my appointment on Tuesday, but instead, it was the nurse from Dr. Zorn's office. Apparently, my CA-125 tumor marker levels came back elevated. The last time I was tested, I was at a 25 or so, but this time I was at a 49. A score of 0-35 is normal. This raises a huge concern for Dr. Zorn, especially since it nearly doubled. There can be many reasons for the increased level, including endometriosis, cysts, as well as cancer, but I have had all of these in the past, and my levels were fine. I'm really freaked out that it has doubled. It is recommended that I return in six weeks for another ultrasound and CA-125 testing. UGH!

I can't say that 2011 is starting off any better than any other year in the past four years. It is quite discouraging, but I will do what I have always done...pick myself up and keep pushing forward. After all, six months from now will be the beginning of my new life.

Wednesday, February 9, 2011
It's Been a Shitty Two Weeks

The last two weeks have been pretty trying. I'm not even sure of where to start.

On Friday, January 28th, I received a Caring Bridge update for my friend, Christine. It was written by her husband, who indicated that Christine was in the hospital, and the doctors were trying to make her comfortable at that point because nothing more could be done. I was devastated, to say the least. I had been emailing and texting her, and she gave no indication that she was not doing well. Several of my cancer cronies and I decided to go to Allegheny General Hospital to see her. I can honestly say that I was not expecting her to be as sick as she was. I knew that things were not good when we got off the elevator and saw all of her family members were sitting in the hallway. It took some time, but we were able to go in to see her. My dear friend was so thin and frail, and we all knew that the end was near. We held each other and never spoke a word. It was so difficult for each of us to see. Here was one of our inner circle of cancer cronies dying. I have been naive in believing this wouldn't happen to my inner circle of cancer cronies.

Tuesday, February 2nd, was a shitty day. I was headed down the stairs to Bud's office to get something for him because he had left in a rush for North Carolina for the birth of his nephew. As I made my way down the stairs, my right foot twisted and before I could catch myself (because I was on the phone with Bud), I went tumbling face-first down my stairs. It was a pretty hard fall, and I hit my head at some point on the way down or when I landed. I didn't make it to work that day because I had lots of bumps and bruises, and probably a slight concussion. Shortly after my fall, I got word that my dear friend, Christine, had passed. UGH!! It was a tough day, and I was all alone.

Friday, February 4th, was the funeral for Christine...it was beautiful and heartbreaking. It was hard to say goodbye. She and I met through a mutual friend after I was diagnosed, and she joined my support group at Gilda's Club. We have laughed and cried together. We have held one another's hand as we traveled this unwanted path. She assured me that one day, I would find someone that loved me for me. Through her relationship with her husband, she has taught me that it is okay to let someone into my world. She was an amazing and inspirational person inside and out. I am angry for so many reasons: because she was so young (she was diagnosed in 2002 at the age of 27) and had so much life yet to live. I'm angry that her husband and daughter are left trying to pick up the pieces of their lives and have to learn to live without her. And I'm angry that she won't be there to celebrate my special day with me.

268

Right after the funeral, I went to the Hillman Cancer Center for another ovarian cancer screening. It was a quick appointment, and I didn't see Dr. Zorn. The ultrasound technician freaked me out a bit. Usually, she tells me that she doesn't see anything of concern. This time, she said that she was writing up a summary for Dr. Zorn. Hmm...I didn't like that. I had the blood test done, and then I was out the door. The nurse said I would hear from them within a week. If my tumor markers are still elevated, they will schedule an appointment at Magee to discuss the next course of action. And as if my Friday couldn't be any more trying, my aunt (my mom's half-sister) emailed me to tell me that she had been diagnosed with liver cancer. WTF???

My monthly friend, Charlie, came to visit on Saturday late in the day. I was okay for most of the day on Sunday, but later in the evening, I started having severe, sharp pains. I was up all night because of the pain. I called the digestive specialist and scheduled a sigmoidoscopy for Tuesday. I was expected to arrive at 7:30 am but didn't get taken in until 10:30 am. It was a long wait, especially considering that I had an IV in my hand that entire time. Bud sat there with me until they wheeled me out to the operating room. The nurses were rather entertaining as we waited for the doctor to arrive, which helped put my mind at ease.

I was out pretty quickly after talking to the doctor. The procedure only took about ten to twenty minutes and then off to recovery I went. The nurses didn't seem irritated with me that I didn't want to wake up, as they usually are. The doctor came in to tell me that they didn't find anything. She mentioned something about trying some medication to treat the symptoms. I was moved to step-down pretty quickly, and then I was out the door to come home. I slept most of the afternoon into the evening. I was up for a little while and then went to bed. I wasn't allowed to drive today because of the anesthesia, so I'm at home again today.

I have been processing the doctor's suggestion that we try some medication to treat the symptoms. I did some research, and most times, they prescribe Lupron. However, there are a few things that concern me about this. 1) I'm not comfortable with taking a medication simply as a band-aid. How can they prescribe something when they don't even know what they are treating? It's not okay to treat only the symptoms and not figure out the cause. 2) Lupron will cause my estrogen levels to first spike and then drop significantly, resulting in menopause-like symptoms. It is not a cure for the endometriosis; it only addresses the symptoms. The side effects of Lupron are less than desirable– weight gain, acne, decreased sexual desire, headaches, generalized pain, vomiting, and on and on and on. No thanks. I have decided that my doctors are wrong. Something is there, but they are missing it. No news is not always good news. My symptoms are consistent with endometriosis...the pain is directly related to my period, and my pain is worse during the heaviest days of my menstrual cycle. Irritable Bowel Syndrome, Crohn's Disease, and other GI issues are not consistent with my symptoms. There is a center in Atlanta that deals specifically with endometriosis so I'm requesting all of my records and sending them down for review. My thought is that we can certainly treat the symptoms, but that doesn't stop whatever it is from growing or getting worse. And in all reality, over the years the symptoms have been getting worse.

Thursday, February 10, 2011
My CA-125 Levels Continue to Climb

Well, I got the dreaded call from my gynecological oncologist's office today a little after 4:00 pm. The nurse called me on my cell phone, which gets pretty poor reception at work, but I got most of what she said. The nurse told me that my tumor markers are now up to 53 and there was something on the sonogram (though I didn't actually hear what she said because my heart dropped, and my cell phone cut out at the same time). Dr. Zorn wants to see me back again for a retest on March 4th. If my tumor markers are still elevated, I will need to meet with my team of doctors to discuss options for surgery. I didn't say anything when she mentioned surgery because I know she isn't the right person to have the discussion with. There will be a discussion of all possible options. I have no intentions of jumping to surgery, for so many different reasons.

I am frustrated, angry, and scared that this is all happening. I should be excited about planning my wedding instead of worrying about the possibility of ovarian cancer. It hardly seems fair, but I suppose life isn't fair, is it? My four-year cancerversary is coming up next month. I want to be celebrating and not preparing for treatments.

Monday, February 8, 2011
Princess Bailey Head Crossed the Rainbow Bridge

Unfortunately, life has continued to deliver blow after blow so far in 2011. The rest of February and March up to this point have continued to be pretty harsh. In mid-February, my ten and a half-year-old cat, Princess Bailey Head, began deteriorating in her health. I took her to the vet on February 14th to run some tests. The vet called me on Wednesday of that week to tell me Bailey had a grade three heart murmur and chronic renal failure. The only options for treatment were a kidney flush followed by continuous injections of fluids, but the odds were stacked against her. When I met with the vet later that day, he explained that my little Princess had some of the highest levels he had seen, and he felt very strongly that she would not respond to the kidney flush.

The only other option was to put her to sleep. I asked if I had to make a decision right then. Thankfully, I did not. I took her home with me after they gave her another injection of fluid and made the decision to wait and see. She wasn't eating, and I couldn't get her to drink much, but there was one thing I knew she would eat– tuna! For the next week, I fed her tuna mixed with water. She was eating it, but the house reeked of fish.

On Monday evening the following week, I started to notice that she had become weaker. She had tried jumping onto the bathroom sink but missed and fell. On Tuesday night, I had given her some tuna and water, which immediately came back up. I made the decision that evening that I would put her down the following day. It was one of the hardest decisions I have ever had to make in my life. That may seem silly to some, but she was my precious baby. She has been with me through everything, including some of the hardest times in my life.

On Wednesday morning, I fed her one last time and then called the vet. Bud and I went down together. We were both a complete mess. They gave her the injection, and I held her in my arms as the sedation took effect. After about 10 minutes, the vet came in and gave her another injection, and she was gone. UGH! I cried for days after and still have my moments; I miss her every day.

Thursday, March 11, 2011
The Blows Just Keep Coming

At the beginning of March, I found out that one of my friends I had met in Las Vegas at the Emerald Dream Ball has been diagnosed with cancer again for the fourth time. It was yet another harsh blow, for her and for all those that love her.

I initially had my ultrasound and CA-125 test scheduled for March 4th at Hillman but had been recruited by my Pink Steel teammates to go to NYC for the filming of a documentary with a photojournalist, Lauren Greenfield, called Beauty CULTure. She has had previous documentaries on HBO– THIN and Girl CULTure. It was a great time, long and exhausting but fun. I got to visit with my cousin Joe and his soon-to-be wife, and we visited with one of Bud's cousins, as well.

On March 8th, I went to Passavant Hospital to get the ultrasound and the CA-125. I showed up at my scheduled time and was promptly taken to the second floor for my test. I told the technician that I did not consume the amount of water that the scheduling person told me to because my doctor's office told me it was not necessary. The technician left the room, and the department head came into the room to tell me that they could not perform the test because I hadn't consumed all the water. I was irritated. I explained over and over that Dr. Zorn, my gynecological oncologist, is only concerned with getting the transvaginal ultrasound, that we never do the abdominal exam. They would not even consider it, telling me repeatedly that this is their protocol. The department head told me several times that she has worked at Passavant for eleven years and that this is the way it has always been. She told me that I could reschedule the appointment. I think that is what made me livid. I looked at her and said, "Do you not understand why I am here? Do you not get that my doctor is concerned about ovarian cancer?" She continued not to care.

My only option was to drink the water and then have the test "when they could get to me." I was even more ticked off that I overheard the one technician talking about me in the hallway with the other technicians as I was walking back to the waiting room. If I didn't have to have the test done, I probably would have told them to shove it (actually I had some other colorful words in my head). Instead of sitting in the waiting room, I went down to have my blood work done, which seemed to take forever, but I'm sure it was because I was angry. I called Dr. Zorn's office and talked with the receptionist. She was pretty hot about the situation, as well. When I returned to the ultrasound suite, I was immediately taken back to be tested. The department head decided to do the ultrasound herself, not sure why that was. The tension in the room could be cut with a knife. It was an awful experience, and I won't be going back to Passavant anytime soon.

The nurse from Dr. Zorn's office called me the following day to let me know the results. I was taken by surprise because it typically takes a week before I hear anything. She told me that she was headed out of town but felt that I needed to know the results. She said that my CA-125 levels are at 28.6. I was initially excited about this because that would mean that they had dropped, but that is not the case. Apparently, Passavant and Hillman do not use the same scale when assessing CA-125 levels. The two scales are not interchangeable, so there is no way to determine how this score correlates to my scores on the tests done at Hillman. The average range on the scale at Passavant is 0-21, so I'm still at an elevated level. They found something on my left ovary that looks like a fluid-filled cyst...nothing to be concerned with but there is something on the right ovary that is more echogenic (this refers to the soundwaves from the ultrasound, so there is something causing it to be louder) and shows more vascularity (this is related to the blood vessels surrounding the ovary). There is something more solid in nature. OKAY...so what does all of that mean? She couldn't tell me anything. She told me she sent the report to Dr. Zorn and that she would probably be calling me the next day to schedule an appointment. Dr. Zorn did call, and she asked that I schedule the appointment at Magee instead of waiting until April to see her at Hillman.

Thursday, March 17, 2011
Having a Heart to Heart with My Gynecological Oncologist

I had an appointment today with Dr. Zorn, my gynecological oncologist. I didn't have to be examined; it was a conversation between the two of us. She shared with me the results of the tests, which is all of what the nurse had said. She told me that there are three types of masses that they can see on ultrasound; fluid-filled cysts (which they know are benign), complex cysts, and solid masses. I have a complex cyst meaning that it is part fluid, part solid. She cannot tell me definitively that it is or isn't cancer. It could also be recurrent endometriosis, but she cannot know unless she removes it. She is recommending that I have my ovaries and fallopian tubes removed but she told me that some other options could be considered. Sometimes Lupron is administered to shut the ovaries down. This would be an injection that could last for either a month or three months. We will monitor my levels while on the Lupron to see if there is any correlation between the two. The Lupron would send me into menopause so the only real difference between it and surgery is that I would be delaying the surgery and it is less permanent. I asked about the possibility of simply going in to remove what they are seeing on the right ovary and to look for more endometriosis, but she didn't seem to think that this was the way to go because there was still too much uncertainty with it. She said that I could opt to have my right ovary removed and leave my left knowing that down the line I may need to have it removed as well. She said I'm between a rock and a hard place right now because she cannot tell me that it isn't cancer.

I asked her about my uterus because we have had previous conversations about removing my ovaries, fallopian tubes, and my uterus. She said they typically do not do that except that in my case, it may be recommended because of the severity of the endometriosis that I had removed in July. She said they may need to do a "sweep" of my pelvic area, which pretty much sounded like scraping the inside of a pumpkin to get rid of everything inside. I asked her about my timeline, as I'm not ready to make a decision right now. She feels that we have some time, but she thinks I need to decide within the next month or so. I told her that I plan to see an endometriosis specialist in Atlanta, and she felt that was a good idea, but hopes that I can get in to see them quickly.

We talked about the surgery, the hospital stay, and the recovery. Dr. Zorn would attempt to do everything through laparoscopic surgery, but there may be a need for larger incisions if things become complicated. Also, if the mass/cyst on my right ovary is cancer, they may have to make a larger incision to determine staging to assess the need for chemotherapy. I'm not sure how I held it all together throughout the entire appointment, but I did. I kind of wished that I had asked Bud to come with me, but I always have to be so damn "strong" and do everything on my own. I was able to get all of my records from all of my appointments with Dr. Zorn, as well as the results from the colonoscopy, sigmoidoscopy, and the surgery in July to send down to Atlanta. I'm also thinking about a second opinion at Cancer Treatment Centers of America.

I'm still trying to process everything. It is a lot to consume. I should be happy right now. I just celebrated my four-year cancerversary on Tuesday, I have my annual Pink Ribbon Princess party on Saturday, and my bridal shower is on Sunday, but I have this hanging over my head. UGH!!

Wednesday, March 23, 2011
Totally Freaking Out

I have been rather stressed since my appointment with Dr. Zorn on March 17th. I didn't sleep Thursday, Friday, or Saturday night. I finally passed out on Sunday evening and was able to sleep through the night. I woke up on Monday feeling very sick, so I stayed home from work. I was able to get in touch with a representative from the Cancer Treatment Centers of America (CTCA) and have my appointment scheduled for April 5th- 7th in Philadelphia. They are flying Bud and me out on Monday evening...yes, they are footing the bill on that. They will provide transportation to and from the airport, to and from the center, and around town. They will put us in a hotel that will cost only seventy-five dollars for the entire duration of my consultation. The assessment is a holistic assessment, so they will look at everything. Chances are that they will do a CT and PET scan, possibly a bone scan, as well as several other assessments. They will also provide me with nutritional support as well, which is something I had sought out previously but was only told to increase my fruit and veggie intake. Before I leave the facility, I will have the results of the tests and a treatment plan in hand.

My experience with CTCA has been enjoyable thus far. The ladies scheduling my appointment, making my travel arrangements, and gathering my medical history have all been very kind.

I am looking forward to my appointment, but I'm a bit nervous. I feel like I'm cheating on my doctors. I trust them with my life, but I would like to know what other options there are for treatment. I am not ready to have surgery to remove my only remaining girlie parts for so many different reasons.

Friday, April 8, 2011
Cancer Treatment Centers of America- Marathon of Tests

This week was my evaluation at Cancer Treatment Centers of America. Bud and I flew to Philadelphia on Monday night and were there until Thursday evening. The first day of the assessment consisted of meeting with several doctors and reviewing my history. I had labs done to check my CA-125 levels, which are up from 53 to 60 at this point. I met with the internist, the medical oncologist, the nutritionist, and many others that I cannot remember at the moment. The appointments with the internist and the medical oncologist were somewhat hard. Bud was in there with me, and up to this point, I have kept him at arm's length from all of this. The medical oncologist asked me why I was so adamantly against having the surgery because my history leads them to believe having surgery would be in my interest. I gave them all of my reasons- not being ready for menopause, not wanting to undergo such a radical and aggressive surgery, and the fact that it makes my decision not to have children final, which has been one of the hardest things for me to come to grips with and one of the things I struggle with every day. I became very emotional when telling them I feel as though I have been cheated and that I have never been married before, and I want to have a healthy relationship with my soon-to-be-husband. As I was crying while sharing this with the doctors, I looked over and saw Bud sitting there with tears in his eyes, too. I don't think he ever knew that was part of my reason for not wanting to do this. The doctors were very understanding and respectful of my reasons for not wanting the surgery. They added on an appointment with the surgical oncologist for the second day after reviewing my records, which bummed me out because I was hoping that surgery would not be a part of the conversation, but that was only wishful thinking. They also added on a CT/PET scan for the following day. We were at the facility from about 9:30 am until 6:00 pm, so it was a long and exhausting day.

The second day of my evaluation started off with the CT/PET scans at 6:45 am followed by consultations with the surgical oncologist, the mind/body/medicine specialist, pastoral care, and several others. My meeting with the surgical oncologist was rather long. We reviewed the results of the CT/PET scans and discussed possible treatment options. I was able to view the scans myself with the doctor, but I was more amused by the fact that my implants are perfectly round and paid little attention to anything else.

The doctor was waiting for the final report from the technician, but he talked about something very slight showing up on my right ovary as "hot." He said that there is some thickening of my uterine lining as well, which is a concern. There was also a "hot" spot on my right breast area. As we were meeting, he rechecked the computer, and the report was there. To his amazement and mine, there was nothing of concern on the ovaries, but the report indicated a spot on the right breast area as a concern. At that point, my head started spinning. I began worrying that all of this time, we have not been doing any scans, and now something is showing up in my breast area. It left me with more questions than answers at that point.

The doctor said that there were many different ways to approach this, but his suggestion would be to remove the right ovary to find out what was going on. He didn't think that leaving it be would be the best decision, but he said the decision was up to me. UGH! It would be so much easier if they could say it is cancer. I would immediately agree with taking it out. There wouldn't be any question in my mind if that were the case. But again, the doctor couldn't tell me if it was cancer and so I felt like I was right back where I was before I had even gone to the center.

I think this appointment was a bit difficult for Bud as well because he had asked the surgical oncologist about harvesting my eggs. We have had the conversation many times before. I told him that they have to pump my body full of estrogen to harvest my eggs, which is not an option because cancer feeds off of the estrogen. On top of that, we would then have to find someone to carry the baby, as I would not be able to do that either because of the estrogen. The doctor told Bud the same things I had and said that it scares him when women in my situation decide to go through with egg harvesting. I was glad that the doctor said the same things I have been telling Bud, but I could see that he was disappointed that the option of one day having our own children is off the table. It broke my heart, and I'm sure it broke his, too. UGH! Our day at the facility ended at about 6:00 pm. I was exhausted again, but we went to the mall and got dinner there rather than eating at the facility (which is all free for patients and caregivers).

The third day of my evaluation was to consist of follow-up appointments with the internist, medical oncologist, and the nutritionist; however, after the team met in the morning (which they do every day to review each case), they decided to add on an MRI. They called me at 9:24 am and asked me to get there as soon as possible. I had just woken up, so we rushed to pack our bags and get out the door to the center. We arrived around 10:30 am. I wasn't able to get anything for breakfast and was starving. I went oncology clinic to have an IV inserted, but it was taking too long, so they sent me to radiology to have the IV put it and to get the MRI done.

Well, things didn't go so well, and it took me a total of three hours to get the MRI done. Three nurses tried to get an IV in, but all of them failed. They tried the crook of my left elbow once, the crook of my right elbow twice, and both of my hands before giving up. I was getting frustrated and was on the verge of tears. The nurse asked the radiologist if we could do the MRI without the contrast, and he was told to call the medical oncologist. It was indicated that we needed to have the MRI contrast, so I had to get an IV somehow. The chief doctor from ultrasound came in and told me that they could get an IV in my upper arm area (right below my armpit) using ultrasound guidance. He offered to use Lidocaine to numb the area to reduce the pain. Well, they got the IV inserted, but it hurt like hell! I screamed about three times and was sobbing...I mean loud, runny nose kind of SOBBING!

The MRI took about an hour to complete, and then I was off to the rest of my appointments. They didn't want to take out the IV in case the doctors ordered more tests. I was thankful for that, but it was uncomfortable all day. Thank goodness I bought a zip-up hoodie at the mall the day before because I wasn't able to put my shirt back on with the IV where it was. It took a long time to meet with the medical oncologist, and that was making me nervous. I had several other appointments that I had missed because I was waiting to see the medical oncologist, but this appointment was most important. I was tired and freezing, so the nurse put me in a reclining chair and gave me a bunch of warm blankets. I was falling in and out of sleep as we waited.

Finally, after about an hour of waiting, the medical oncologist came in to share the results of the MRI. She said that nothing showed up in the chest area or the pelvic area!! YAY!! She said that contrary to what the surgical oncologist (and the rest of the team) thought and said yesterday, there is no reason for us to jump to surgery right now. She would like for me to follow-up either with them or with Dr. Zorn in six to eight weeks. I'm clear...there is no cancer! I was so excited, but so tired and ready to go home. So as of right now, I will not be having surgery. Yippee! I was stressing over this because I wasn't sure when I would be able to squeeze in surgery with the end of the school year and my wedding around the corner.

I met with the nutritionist again. She seemed pleased with my diet. She gave me some literature on sugar and cancer, soy and cancer, and Vitamin D supplement because I am now deficient even though my last test showed that I wasn't. I am not shocked by this, considering Pittsburgh has no sun. We were headed from that appointment to the airport, but I still needed to have the IV taken out. The medical oncologist sent over a nurse to remove it. She was taken aback by the location of the IV and felt awful for all that I had gone through to get the darn thing put in. She even gave me a secret for the next time. The nurse was even more taken aback by the size of the IV. Apparently, the doctor had put in a six-inch IV rather than the usual inch. She immediately hid it behind her back so that I could not see it, but Bud made a comment on the size of it. The nurse said it probably went all the way up into my armpit. EW!! Bud and I ate dinner at the center, and then we were off to the airport. We were both thrilled that we had come to the center and that everything is clear!

I was impressed with the Cancer Treatment Centers of America. The approach to cancer treatment is holistic and integrative, which is very important in my opinion. It is a different feel and a different atmosphere compared to the hospitals where I have been treated to this point. I met so many different people being treated there that were told from their doctors at home there was nothing more that could be done and then they went to CTCA, they were given hope and their treatment was continued. I was amazed to learn that CTCA will send people to Europe for additional treatment if they cannot do anything more in the United States or sometimes, they will bring in doctors from Europe if the patient cannot travel. I cannot say enough positive things about CTCA, honestly.

Of course, I'm now in a position of trying to figure out where I want to continue receiving my care. I love my current gynecological oncologist, Dr. Zorn, but there has always been a push for me to remove my ovaries, which is something I have always struggled with. CTCA is more understanding of my concerns and will not jump to surgery without looking at everything! I called my Dr. Zorn to share the results but have not yet heard from anyone at this point.

I am so thankful and excited that whatever was on my right ovary is either gone or not anything of concern! No surgery for me. I may have an "I'm not having surgery party" to celebrate!!!

Saturday, April 9, 2011
Marathon Testing All for Nothing?

Yesterday, I made the call to Dr. Zorn's office to share with them the results of the evaluation done at the CTCA and to find out how they would like to proceed from here. I didn't get through, but the nurse called me back around 4:30 pm. I missed her call but returned her call and got through to her before she left for the day. I told her that I went for a second opinion (never said where I went) and had a CT/PET scan and an MRI done, all of which indicated that my ovaries are normal. I told her that they didn't say the mass was gone, but it wasn't showing up as anything of concern. She asked if I had a transvaginal ultrasound repeated, and I told her that I had not.

She then told me that the tests done at CTCA are not sensitive enough to detect ovarian cancer and are not the tests they prefer to use when screening or diagnosing. I went from high to low in a matter of seconds. I was confused by that, and if it is indeed the case, I don't understand how it is that in a world where we can clone, we do not have the technology to detect ovarian cancer before it becomes deadly! It is all very frustrating. So, at the end of the day, it sounds (from the nurse) as though Dr. Zorn will still recommend surgery, but someone will be calling me to let me know how Dr. Zorn wants to proceed with the new information.

UGH!!!

Friday, April 15, 2011
Between a Rock and a Hard Place

I have an appointment with my gynecological oncologist, Dr. Zorn, on Thursday, April 21st, to discuss the results of the tests from CTCA. I'm preparing myself that her recommendation will still be for me to have surgery. I may ask her to conduct another transvaginal ultrasound and to recheck my CA-125 levels. If need be, I will get a third opinion. I feel like I'm between a rock and a hard place with the different recommendations from my doctors and CTCA. I have been emailing my medical oncologist, Dr. Puhalla, about the situation since I was in Philly. She has helped answer some of my questions and is more than willing to meet with me to discuss things.

Monday, May 2, 2011
She Isn't Even My Doctor

I met with Dr. Zorn, my gynecological oncologist, on April 21st, to discuss the results from CTCA and her recommendations. I had to go down to Magee to see Dr. Zorn because she was not at Hillman that day. I was taken aback pretty quickly. The nurse seemed to be annoyed with me because she kept asking me the reason for my visit, and all I could tell her was that we were discussing the second opinion. I guess that wasn't good enough for her. She then became annoyed with me when she handed me a gown and told me to get undressed, and I said there was no reason for that. Dr. Zorn has never done an internal exam on me. I asked the nurse to check to see if it was necessary, and she returned shortly to say that I did, in fact, need to get undressed. I sat waiting for a few minutes before a doctor that I don't know came in and started having a conversation with me about where I am with the surgery. I can only imagine the look on my face because I was in shock that this was how she started the conversation. I asked her if she had even looked at the results from CTCA. She had but indicated that PET/CT and MRI scans are not the golden-standard tools used for detecting ovarian cancer. She then asked me if my medical oncologist had seen the results given the hot spot on my right breast area. She seemed to make this out to be more of an issue than CTCA had, which freaked me out.

After our short conversation about the results from CTCA, she returned to the surgery conversation. I told her that I have no interest in having the surgery, but I certainly would do whatever is within my best interest. However, that being said, there had better be some hard data to support my need for surgery. What the doctor said next almost sent me over the edge. She told me that if I have no intentions of having children, then why even bother to keep my ovaries and that most people follow the guidelines set forth for BRCA1 and 2 carriers. At that point, I felt like I wasn't being treated as an individual...I was simply a number, just another cancer patient. I couldn't hold back my tears. I told her that I am not most people. I am an individual and that I have so MANY reasons that I do not want to have this surgery. I think it finally took my crying for her to stop with the questioning. I was so irritated when she left the room.

After several minutes, this doctor returned with Dr. Zorn. We had the conversation about ultrasound versus PET/CT scans and MRI. Dr. Zorn also said that ultrasound is more sensitive in evaluating the ovaries. We then had a conversation about surgery. I very bluntly asked her if her recommendation for me is to move forward with surgery despite the results from CTCA. I don't remember if she said yes or no, but she did say that the tests done at CTCA were encouraging. She asked me why I was so opposed to having this surgery. Finally, after four years of meeting with her, I had a very candid and real conversation with her about it. I told her that there are so many reasons that I would avoid having this surgery if at all possible. I explained that every single day, I struggle with my not having children and that having my ovaries removed makes that decision final. I'm not sure that I can handle that emotionally. Physically, I'm sure I will be fine, but emotionally, I will be a complete mess.

I also told her that I'm not ready to be in menopause at the age of 36. She asked me about the side effects of Tamoxifen, which are very much like being in menopause except that I'm still having my periods. Her comment to me was that if I'm already in pseudo-menopause, what is the difference? As I continued to try talking through my tears, I explained to her that there is definitely a difference between having menopausal-like symptoms and actually being in menopause. I'm not ready to be in full-blown menopause.

I explained to her that I am about to be married for the first time in my life and as a part of my marriage, I would like to have a healthy intimate relationship with my soon-to-be husband. I hope that in a year, I can go off of the Tamoxifen, which has completely squelched all desire for any intimate relations. I want to have a healthy relationship with my husband for a few years before I make the decision to have my ovaries removed. I explained that Bud came along in the middle of all of this (and my menopausal-like symptoms). I find it unfair to him and unfair to me that I have absolutely no desire! I think that it finally sunk in with them why I struggle with this so much, and that wasn't even all of my reasons for not wanting to have the surgery. I told her that I was less than ninety days from my wedding and surgery doesn't fit in anywhere from now until then. She said we don't need to jump to surgery at this point and also said she is comfortable with a "wait and see" approach. She suggested that I go in for my next appointment in August. I asked about doing the CA-125 tests every 6 months instead of every year, but she didn't seem to think we needed to do that unless there was something on the ultrasound that would suggest otherwise.

So, I'm not having surgery before my wedding, which makes me very happy. I haven't done anything with the wedding for the past three months because I have been stressed out over all of this. Let's hope everything falls into place.

Thursday, June 2, 2011
Here We Go Again

I went to see my medical oncologist, Dr. Puhalla, today for my now tri-annual appointment. My appointment was scheduled for 1:30 pm and, for the first time, I was actually ten minutes early. To my dismay, I sat in the waiting room for a very long time before I was called back to have my vitals checked (I have lost four pounds, by the way). I returned to the waiting room and after another twenty minutes was taken back to an exam room at 2:37 pm. UGH! I waited another ten minutes before the nurse came in. I have to admit I don't enjoy her as much as I enjoyed the other nurse. She isn't warm and fuzzy, and she asks me some of the silliest questions. We reviewed what has gone on since my last appointment. She seemed to be clueless about the whole ovary thing. We talked a bit about CTCA and the results from the PET scan that indicated a "hot spot" on my right chest wall. I gave her copies to give to Dr. Puhalla. I told her I was a bit freaked out by my appointment with Dr. Zorn because the doctor I had seen before Dr. Zorn seemed to be much more concerned than the folks at CTCA.

Honestly, I didn't look at the report to know what it said. I read through it as I was sitting in the waiting room– probably not the best idea right before my appointment. The PET scan revealed a single focus of abnormal hypermetabolism– differential diagnosis early infiltrating muscle metastasis versus muscle strain or other traumatic/inflammatory non-neoplastic etiology. In plain English: they questioned whether it is cancer recurrence or a strain, but nothing confirmed either one. So pretty much, we don't know.

Following the discussion with the nurse and having an exam, I waited for Dr. Puhalla. She came in, asked how I was doing, and immediately asked me why I didn't tell her about the results of the PET scan. I was honest with her and told her that I didn't even think anything of it because the folks at CTCA didn't seem concerned. I also shared that I hadn't actually read the report until now. Shame on me! She said that an SUV (standard uptake value) of 2.5 is considered high and of concern. My SUV from the PET in April was 5. She said that there can be some things that pop up on a PET following breast surgery but considering that I'm almost three years out from my last breast surgery, she is concerned. UGH! UGH! UGH! She asked me if I wanted to do the PET before or after the wedding. Maybe I'm crazy, but I said before, if it is metastatic breast cancer, I would want to know right now and start treatment ASAP, regardless of the wedding. I'm not quite sure how well I will handle this before the wedding if it turns out to be the worst-case scenario, but I know that if I wait until after the wedding and find out that it is metastatic cancer, I will be really pissed off at myself for waiting.

286

We talked about stopping Tamoxifen next July– it will be five years!! Woo Hoo!! She recommended that we consider an aromatase inhibitor for ovarian suppression (medical menopause), but I talked with her about my feelings on that. I brought up the same issues that I did with Dr. Zorn, and Dr. Puhalla was also very understanding. She is okay with letting me go off the Tamoxifen and waiting a few years before starting another medication or having my ovaries removed. YAY! That was at least something positive. She did the exam and seemed to be concerned with the "dimpling" that I have on the lower half of my right implant, which has gotten bigger but said that overall, she didn't have any concerns with the physical exam.

The PET scan is not scheduled yet. I have to wait for someone to call me with a date and time. I see my surgical oncologist for my one-year follow-up next Tuesday. I'm hoping the PET scan can be scheduled for the following week.

Here we go again...

Friday, June 17, 2011
Broken Heart

On Tuesday, June 13th, I went to Magee to have a follow-up CT/PET scan to the one done at CTCA in April. By most accounts, it was pretty routine and took a few hours from beginning to end. Not sure how much radioactive dye, contrast, and iodine they put into my body, but it made me sick. I was totally wiped out the rest of the day, and I felt like at any moment fluid was going to come spewing out of my body from either end. Eventually, it did. Pleasant, I know.

I called Dr. Philla's office today to get the results. The nurse called back to find out where I had the test done because the only one on file was from April, and of course, I missed this call. UGH! I called back to tell her that it was done at Magee. I waited and waited and waited until I could no longer. I called again and asked for someone to please call me back on my cell phone. Dr. Puhalla finally called as I was almost home. I was a bit nervous when I heard her voice because I knew that meant something wasn't right. She said that the results of the CT/PET were okay. There is some uptake (a "hot spot") that continues to show up on the right side. Again, it could be several things causing this– muscle activity, radiation, or metastatic breast cancer– but the techs were not overly concerned with it, so that was encouraging. She wants to repeat the CT/PET in three or four months. Not great, but not the worst thing I could have heard.

She then tells me that they were a bit concerned with my heart, though. WHAT? She said that my aorta (the main artery going into the heart) was dilated and there is some enlargement of my heart. I think my heart stopped at that point. So, I have to go see a cardiologist and have an echocardiogram (sonogram of my heart) done. Really? Come on, can't I get a flipping break here?! I told her that I had been to my primary care physician in the winter months and when he listened to my heart, he said there was something suspicious, so they ran an EKG which turned out to be fine. I believe he said there was something minor on the EKG but nothing to be concerned with. Off to the cardiologist for more tests. Yippee! Isn't it flipping fabulous to be me! She said that there were cysts on both of my ovaries with no uptake in either one, but there was some uptake in my endometrium. GRR!!

I know that I should be happy that I wasn't told I have metastatic breast cancer, or at least that they cannot confirm that I do at this point, but I'm frustrated! This year has been exceptionally hard for me. I mean, the last four years have been hard, but this year may possibly take the cake! Even during my initial diagnosis and all of the surgeries, radiation, etc., I don't think I have been to the doctors as much as I have been in the past six months. I'm tired and worn out. I feel like I have nothing left in me to keep going. I will, but I'm SO tired! Whatever happened to "get through this year and everything will be back to normal" that someone said to me back in 2007? Gosh, I wish I could remember who that person was. It has never happened to me.

Dr. Puhalla asked me if I wanted to wait until after the wedding to get this all scheduled and of course, I do not. I am one of those people who needs to know now what is going on, and if it is something that needs to be treated, we can just do it. She said we could probably get it scheduled for next week sometime, so I guess I will have to wait and see what happens then.

Wednesday, June 30, 2011
My Beating Heart

I went to Magee to meet with the cardiologist on Wednesday, June 29th. I have come to realize that I now have a doctor on every floor in that hospital except for level two, which is the maternity floor. Sadly, that still breaks my heart. My friend Amy came with me to keep me company at the appointment. I'm sure she had nothing better to do for a few hours! I was actually early, so I had to wait for about a half-hour before I was taken back for the echocardiogram– using ultrasound to capture images of the heart. I was able to view the screen the entire time they were conducting the echocardiogram. The nurse seemed to be a bit frustrated because she couldn't find my heart– those damn foobies were in the way. After several attempts, she finally found it. I must admit that seeing my heart on the screen humored me. It looked like a little monster. When I said that, the nurse looked at me like I was crazy. I will chalk that up to her lack of personality. After capturing the images from the middle of my chest, she moved over to my side. I wasn't expecting any pain, but the placement of the wand was right on my ribs, and she kept pushing it back and forth. Just when I thought it was over, she asked if her student could capture some images. I agreed, but of course, she only captured images from my side. I thought for sure I might have a bruise from it.

I returned to the waiting room. After about twenty minutes, I was taken back to a room to meet with the Cardiologist. The nurse came in and asked several questions and then informed me that she would be doing an EKG. I had to get undressed again to have that done. I'm not sure why they didn't do both tests one after the other, but whatever. The doctor came in, and I'm sure he probably thinks I'm crazy. He was laughing the entire time. My humor was in full force that day because I was nervous and didn't know what else to do. We talked about my family history of heart disease on my mother's side and my current situation. He said that I'm on the high end of the normal range, right on the cusp of what would be considered abnormal with dilation of 3.8 cm. He indicated that he is not overly concerned with it at this point. He then went into a long explanation about having a dilated aorta and an enlarged heart. He said I should come back in for another exam in two or three years. He said he would be more concerned if the dilation became larger over that time. I asked him how much it had grown from the scan done at CTCA to the one done at Magee because I knew it was different. He looked at me kind of funny and then admitted he hadn't looked at the scan from Magee. Oops! He reviewed it and said that he still isn't too concerned with it but that I should make an appointment to see him after my next CT Scan, which will be in September/October. I shared that I had been experiencing chest pains while dragon boating, so he ordered a stress test. I offered to run in my bare feet so that I could get it done that day, but there were no openings, which meant I had to return the following day for the stress test.

Tuesday, July 12, 2011
Stress Test: Passed

On Thursday, July 7th, I went for a stress test. I wasn't allowed to eat anything after 10:00 am, so I ate at 9:50 am. I was able to drink fluids until the time of my appointment at 1:00 pm. I arrived a little early and was taken back pretty quickly. Two technicians were working with me again, but not the same ones from the day before. These ladies were awesome. They thought I was the cutest thing ever. They told me this, so it must be true. One prepped me for the stress test while the other was set up the monitor to do an echocardiogram before and after the test.

I didn't realize that I would have to be set up with an IV to do the stress test. I explained that I'm a tough stick, but she assured me she would get it the first time. She examined both of my arms and then said, "You really are tough. You have no veins." I laughed and told her I had already warned her. She made her first attempt on my left arm. She couldn't get the vein and tried digging around for it. It was becoming painful, and finally, I told the nurse, "you should go ahead and take that out." She laughed and then took it out. She looked at my right arm and realized that it would be just as tricky but made an attempt anyway. No luck on that side either. She decided that instead of trying to find a vein and keep poking me, she would call the IV Team to get one. She apologized over and over again that she wasn't able to get me. I told her I'm glad she stopped because I would hate to be bruised for my wedding. She was stunned and said, "Why in the world are you doing this fifteen days before your wedding?" I explained that I dragon boat and I run, so I want to make sure that I'm okay to do both of those. The Cardiologist came in to see if we were ready and she told him that they couldn't get an IV in me, so he said to do it without. This is not their typical protocol, so they weren't sure how to do it. Apparently, this had only happened one other time. They set me up to do the stress test without the IV...YAY!!!

The technician did the echocardiogram before the test, and then I was ready to go on the treadmill. The Cardiologist said he wanted me to go for at least nine minutes. I wasn't able to wear my sports bra. I was concerned that the foobies would hurt if I were forced to run. I power walked the entire time and went to twelve minutes. I had the technicians and doctor laughing as I was on the treadmill, as well. After twelve minutes, they hit the big red stop button and hustled me over to the gurney to do the echocardiogram. The Cardiol looked at it and said everything is all good. I am cleared to exercise! Woo Hoo!! I will go back to see the doctor after my next CT Scan and see what comes of it then. He assured me that my heart is not going to burst.

As life goes these days, I haven't been able to run because my treadmill broke and I haven't had time to get out in the boat because my nights and weekends have been consumed with wedding stuff. I can hardly believe that I am now only four days away from my wedding. It has been a long, tough road since January to get to this point. There were so many months that went by that I did nothing with the wedding because of something with my health. There were times I wasn't quite sure if it was going to happen at all. I feel as though I'm in a better place right now, though I have been experiencing constant aching pain in my who-ha for the past few weeks. I will deal with that after the wedding. I'm ready to have one night where I will be surrounded by my friends and family in celebration of this next chapter in my life.

Thursday, October 13, 2011
Life Changes so Fast

Wow! I cannot believe I haven't written in my journal for three months.

Gosh, so much has happened in that time. Of course, the biggest thing is that I am now a married woman. I am now MRS. ADAMS!! The wedding was absolutely beautiful. Everything went as planned except for the breast cancer cake. I never wanted a breast cancer cake. I had a great time and never wanted it to end.

Since the wedding, I have been in to see my plastic surgeon– Dr. Gimbel, my gynecological oncologist– Dr. Zorn, and my medical oncologist– Dr. Puhalla. I also had another CT/PET Scan. My plastic surgeon indicated that everything looks good with the foobies, so that was a pretty quick and easy appointment. I went for a follow-up with my gynecological oncologist, Dr. Zorn, on August 19th. My CA-125 levels continue to be elevated, and there was something on one of my ovaries. Dr. Zorn recommended that I have a retest of both, which I did at the end of September/beginning of October. My CA-125 levels are still elevated. I have to go back in another month to have them checked. If they continue to be elevated, Dr. Zorn said we will discuss, "where we go from there."

My ovaries looked good, and there were no concerns so, for right now, I don't have to repeat the pelvic ultrasound. I had a repeat CT/PET Scan at the end of September that showed some uptake/activity on the right chest wall and in my uterus. Dr. Puhalla seems to think the uptake on the chest wall is related to the mastectomy and the uptake in the uterus is connected to my menstrual cycle, but we will continue to monitor in case that is not what it is. I have to go back in six months for a follow-up CT/PET scan. I'm glad they moved the scans to six months rather than every three because all the crap they make me put into my body makes me sick for a few days. Quite unpleasant, I must say.

In talking with Dr. Zorn, she indicated she is concerned with the continued pain I have been experiencing. While the pain is constant and varies in severity and intensity, I am tolerating it. She feels I need to consider the impact of the pain on my daily activities. At some point, I need to make the decision to have a pelvic sweep. Usually, during this part of the conversation, I start to hear the teacher from Charlie Brown talking. There is a possibility that the endometriosis has returned. Yes, I did have surgery in July 2010 to remove a significant amount of it, so I will contact Dr. Mansuria to see if he thinks I should come back in for a visit. I was reminded that the only way to stop it from returning is to have everything removed. I have read information that suggests otherwise, so I'm not sure.

I took a break from the Pink Steel dragon boating team, so I can focus on the new life I am creating with my hubby, to spend more time with my family, and to work toward achieving my career goals. I never thought I would see the day that I would take a break because I love dragon boating so much, but I cannot make the time commitment necessary to be the best athlete I can be for myself, my team, or my coach.

Bud and I traveled to Cincinnati to see the SCARProject at the beginning of October. He was deeply touched by the exhibit and found it quite emotional.

Monday, March 12, 2012
Five-Year Cancerversary

On Thursday, March 15, 2007, I received the phone call at work that turned my life completely upside down, and this year on Thursday, March 15th, I will be celebrating my five-year cancerversary!! Can you believe it?!?! It seems almost surreal as it feels like it was just yesterday that I was diagnosed. It is both exciting and emotional at the same time. I have grown so much through all of this and have gained so much more than I could have ever imagined. It's hard to imagine how one's life can be positively changed by cancer unless you have walked that journey.

I haven't been to any of my doctors since the end of last year. I am back to being monitored every six months for any potential of ovarian cancer, and we are now doing CT/PET scans every six months as well. In May, I will see my surgical oncologist, Dr. Ahrendt, for the last time. This November should be the last time I have to see my radiation oncologist, Dr. Beriwal, as well. It is scary to think I won't have all the watchful eyes keeping tabs on me.

I continue to have pelvic pain, as well as pain in my rectum, which we think may be a recurrence of endometriosis even though I had surgery in July 2010 to remove it. I meet with Dr. Mansuria on April 3rd to discuss the surgery options, as surgery is the only treatment option now. We will talk about conducting some additional tests of my abdominal lining to make sure there is no active cancer there, as it is rare for endometriosis to return so quickly. He did indicate that the Tamoxifen could possibly be the culprit here, but there is very little research to show the link between Tamoxifen and growth of endometriosis.

Though the past five years haven't exactly been easy, I'm looking forward to the next five years, the next five after that, and many more after that. I realize that my cancer journey may never be over, and that cancer is something I could be faced with again merely because of the BRCA2 mutation, but it is something I am learning to accept. I refuse to live my life in fear and am taking every day for what it is.

I will simply continue to laugh often, live sincerely, and love deeply.

Thursday, April 19, 2012
Another Surgery

I went to see Dr. Mansuria, my gynecological specialist, on April 3rd. The visit was pretty short and sweet. We discussed my symptoms and my only option for treatment for what we think may be endometriosis, which is surgery. I had expected that we would wait until July for me to have the surgery since I will end my five years of Tamoxifen, but he seems to have some type of urgency to schedule me for the first available slot. Ok!?!? We discussed the different surgical options. I explained that I would first like to try the laparoscopic surgery first and see if being off the tamoxifen makes a difference before I jump to a full pelvic sweep. We talked about my emotional struggles with the pelvic sweep. While I appreciate what he does, there is so much more to it than just doing the surgery...from my end. He understands that I have done lots of research and have explored the different options. He supports me in whatever decision I make. He told me that he always enjoys talking with me because it helps to keep him grounded. That was nice to hear.

He indicated that while the symptoms are the same as what I was having previously, there is a possibility that it isn't endometriosis but something else. During the surgery, he plans to do a water test where they will fill my belly with water, jiggle it around, and look for any cancer cells. If anything comes back cancerous, the game plan changes. More than likely, this means I will have to undergo the full pelvic sweep...no more ovaries, no more uterus, no more fallopian tubes... just emptiness, completely empty!

Dr. Mansuria said he would have the nurse call me with a date for the surgery, which will be done at Passavant Hospital. I wasn't expecting it to be so soon, but they called that afternoon and had April 26th open for surgery. My schedule at work is already pretty full through the end of April and Bush is coming to the Pittsburgh on April 25th, so I asked for another date. I am scheduled to go in May 8th. I have a two-week recovery if the surgery only involves removing endometriosis. If I end up having to do the full pelvic sweep, it will be a 6-8 week recovery time.

Friday, May 4, 2012
It's Hard to Say Goodbye

I had my six-month follow-up CT/PET Scan on April 17th. Somehow, I have forgotten to schedule an appointment with my medical oncologist, Dr. Puhalla, and haven't seen her since September. Since I didn't have a follow-up appointment scheduled, I called the office to get the results of the testing. At this point, everything with my chest, uterus, and heart are stable, and no changes were noted. YAY!

I had my final appointment with my surgical oncologist, Dr. Ahrendt, on May 1st. It was a bitter sweet appointment for both of us, I think. It seems so surreal that five years ago, on May 3rd, I underwent my bilateral mastectomy. She examined my foobies and continues to be pleased with the outcome. She is surprised that I still have a "bump" where my right latissimus muscle was used to rebuild my right breast. She had expected that it would have diminished over time, but that hasn't been the case.

We talked about the next steps in my treatment from here. I shared with her that I plan to go off the Tamoxifen for a few years and then consider having the full pelvic sweep. She asked what my medical oncologist would like to do for treatment. I shared with her that Dr. Puhalla and I have discussed putting me on Lupron to put me into medical menopause. I explained all of my concerns and reasons for not wanting to take the Lupron, and she understood. Dr. Ahrendt also feels that at some point, my quality of life needs to be a priority rather than continued cancer treatments. She recommended that I talk with my medical oncologist to determine what the benefits would be of being placed on Lupron. Let's say that the Tamoxifen reduces my risk of recurrence of breast cancer by ten percent and then taking Lupron reduces it by another two to five percent. Is it worth it? I couldn't agree more!

I will miss seeing Dr. Ahrendt and having her watchful eye over me. It was hard to say goodbye to her but after 5 years, it is time.

Friday, May 11, 2012
Post-Surgery Update

On Tuesday, May 8th, I underwent laparoscopic surgery for possible removal of what we expected to be a recurrence of endometriosis. I had to be at the hospital by 5:15 am. I was taken back to pre-op relatively quickly. Bud wasn't allowed to be with me for about an hour. Considering that I had been up most of the night, it was an opportunity for me to take a nap. I most of my prep was finished before Bud got there. Within forty-five minutes, I was being wheeled off for my seventh surgery in five years. The operation only took an hour, and I was in the recovery room by 8:30 am. I was in recovery much longer than I had ever been before- six hours. When I woke up, I was in so much pain. I asked for some pain medication, which was administered via my IV and was out again for some time. I woke up moaning and groaning again that I was in pain and was given more medication to control the pain. I do remember telling the nurse that I had dropped my pen. She told me that I must have been dreaming because I don't have a pen; I had undergone surgery and was in recovery. Quickly after that, I was knocked out again. The third time I woke up, I told the nurse that I was nauseous. She offered to give me something to take care of that but said, "every time I give you something, it knocks you out." I declined the medication. She asked me if I felt as though I could get out of bed. I gave her a sideways look. She said, "Yeah, I don't think so either." The nurse sat me up some and gave me ginger ale and crackers. It took me about an hour to eat one packet of crackers. I was still feeling nauseous and was still in a lot of pain but was trying to push through it to work my way to step-down recovery. Another nurse told me that I will likely end up staying much longer if I don't take the nausea medication through the IV and sleep for another hour. I finally gave in and asked for the medication. I called Bud to tell him that it would be a little while longer in recovery. Unfortunately, I ended up being out for about two hours.

While in the recovery room, my blood pressure dropped. The nurse began pushing fluids through my IV to help get it back up. When I woke up again, I felt so much better. I wasn't a hundred percent, but I thought I could go to step-down recovery. I had to pee so bad because of all the fluids being pushed into my system. I expected to get up and go to the bathroom, but I was brought a bedpan instead. As much as I didn't want to do it, I had to because I was about to pee the bed! Gosh, I hate being so vulnerable and right at that moment, I was. I couldn't use the toilet on my own. UGH! After going to the bathroom for what seemed like ten minutes, I was cleaned up and then wheeled over to step-down recovery. Bud was able to join me shortly after. He told me that the news was good but not so good.

Dr. Mansuria didn't find any cancer on my ovaries, but he also didn't find any endometriosis either. I was stunned! I'm completely baffled as to what could be going on with me. I heard Dr. Mansuria out in the hallway and asked if he would be able to come and talk to me. He told me he removed a cyst but felt it was likely benign. He said that we would have the results of the water test back in about a week. I am guessing this is to determine if there is cancer in my stomach lining, which can present as something else. I told Dr. Mansuria that he had ruined my day because I am now back at square one with no answers. He told me that sometimes people merely have pain. Although I didn't say anything, I don't believe that some people simply have this kind of pain. It is not normal, and I will not accept that as a reason. He told me that the only option for relief is to have the full pelvic sweep but also said that there is only a seventy percent chance that my symptoms will cease. UGH!! I think I lost all hope right then and there.

After talking with Dr. Mansuria, I was ready to go...or at least, I just wanted to go. I was still in pain but was told that if I were given more pain medication, I would have to be held for at least twenty minutes. That, of course, would actually mean another hour because even the Vicodin would knock me out. I sucked it up and was released at 3:30 pm. We went to fill my scripts for pain medication and headed home.

I slept all day on Tuesday, Wednesday, and Thursday. I stopped taking the Vicodin on Thursday and am now using the Ibuprofen. Dr. Mansuria called on Wednesday to say that the cyst was benign. Now I have to wait for the results of the water test. It is all pretty frustrating. I feel so hopeless and helpless that I still have no answers. I had expected for this to be a recurrence of endometriosis, but Dr. Mansuria did say that it is very uncommon for it to return so quickly. I'm not sure what my plans are from here. I will wait to see what comes from the water test and go from there.

I came across this article yesterday, and it struck home with me as to why I continue to be resistant to having the pelvic sweep (one of the reasons, anyway). While it will definitely reduce my chances of developing ovarian cancer, it only diminishes my chance of getting other cancers.

http://www.thejewishweek.com/features/all_she_wrote/risky_surgical_business

Monday, May 14, 2012
Cancer is Always in The Back of My Mind

I have been pretty anxious waiting to hear the results of the water test...hopefully that news will come tomorrow or Wednesday. I think part of me is nervous because there is always a possibility that it is cancer. What worries me the most is that I have been having these symptoms and the pain since August 2007...almost five years. We have done test after test after test and have found nothing, but it makes me wonder...have they been doing the right tests? I'm not sure.

It is rare for one to develop cancer in the lining of the stomach but let's be honest, it is rare to have the BRCA mutation, it is rare to have had the complications I had with the radiation and the implant...rare has always seemed to be my running theme here. I have been reading up on peritoneal cancer (cancer that develops in the peritoneum- a thin, delicate sheet that lines the inside wall of the abdomen and covers the uterus and extends over the bladder and rectum) and here is what I have found...

Women who are at an increased risk of developing ovarian cancer, particularly due to the BRCA1 and BRCA2 genetic mutations, also are at increased risk for peritoneum cancer (isn't that lovely...and yes, this means that even if I have the full pelvic sweep, I am still at risk for this type of cancer). Symptoms of peritoneum cancer can be very vague and difficult to spot.

The symptoms of this type of cancer can mimic those of ovarian cancer. There is no effective method to test for this type of cancer. Internal ultrasounds, as used for ovarian cancer detection, are just as ineffective for peritoneal cancer as it is ovarian cancer. The CA-125 test is another method used but again, not always effective. However, the one thing I read that scared me is that an increase in CA-125 can be a red flag (if you remember last year my CA-125 went from 25 to 49 and had continued to increase, which prompted all of the concern and my marathon ovarian cancer screenings).

I know that something is not right with my body, whether it be cancer or something else. I know that it is not typical to experience the level of pain that I have daily. At times, the intensity of the pain takes my breath away and stops me in my tracks. I cannot even begin to believe that this is normal, and I cannot accept that I have to live this way. I remember one of the doctors at CTCA telling me to keep on top of these symptoms because they are not normal.

What sucks right now is not only do I have the pain from the surgery and a blood blister that burst near one of my incisions but also the pain that I

300

have always had. The ibuprofen eases the pain slightly, but unless I'm completely knocked out, nothing even touches the pain in my rectum. I had taken a Vicodin last night and still even with that, I was up all night in pain.

I'm so tired of being sick and tired all of the time...and even more tired of always being in pain.

Tuesday, May 15, 2012
No Cancer!

I spoke with Dr. Mansuria today regarding the tests and the surgery. Everything came back benign...the cyst he had taken off my ovary and the test they had done to see if there was any cancer in my abdominal lining. I am relieved that there is no cancer, but I'm still frustrated that we still do not know what is causing the pain. He said that he didn't see any muscle spasms in the pelvic area while doing the surgery but thinks that maybe we can try pelvic physical therapy. Of course, the conversation always has and will go back to my doing the full pelvic sweep, and Dr. Mansuria feels that it is something to be considered from a pain standpoint and a BRCA2 mutation standpoint, but he understands my hesitation with the procedure. He reiterated that he cannot guarantee it will stop my pain, and while seventy percent may sound good, there is still a thirty percent chance I could have the same pain. I laughed at him and told him that didn't seem all that good to me. I have my four-week follow-up with him on June 19th, and we will discuss the physical therapy then.

Thursday, June 7, 2012
I Just Want Some Normalcy

I had my six-month follow-up with Dr. Zorn, my gynecological oncologist, on June 8th. Nothing showed up on the pelvic sonogram other than a few cysts, which is very typical for me. My CA-125 levels continue to increase, so I am scheduled to return in September for another CA-125 blood test. We talked at great length about my five years of Tamoxifen coming to an end and my decision not to take an aromatase inhibitor as suggested by my medical oncologist, Dr. Puhalla. We discussed the risks of not doing anything, which I am well aware of, but I do believe that at some point, the quality of my life has to outweigh the cancer treatments. Right now, I want to take a break for a few years and be "normal" again. We also talked about my feelings of abruptly throwing myself into medical menopause and how I feel that it will be very traumatic for my body. I whole-heartedly believe that our bodies prepare us for that life change. I prefer to let it happen naturally. There are risks involved in that, and I am well aware of those risks. Again, the quality of my life takes precedence! I asked about the monitoring that would occur following the removal of my remaining girly parts, and she said that I would still be followed as there are continued risks for cancer in other areas. That, at least, gave me some level of comfort to know that I won't be "let go."

Thursday, June 21, 2012
No Leaking Foobies, I Hope

On June 19th, I had an MRI done to check the implants for any leaks before seeing Dr. Gimbel, my plastic surgeon, in August. The MRI was fairly uneventful other than my right arm going completely numb and the technician becoming impatient with me. I was excited that I didn't have to get an IV or drink anything! YAY! And of course, that everything looks clear on the MRI. I went from the MRI to my follow-up with Dr. Mansuria, my gynecological specialist. It was a very brief appointment. He was pleased with how everything has healed. We discussed the pelvic physical therapy but agreed to wait until I am finished with Tamoxifen to see if that has any impact on the pain I have been experiencing.

Tuesday, June 26, 2012
Stable CT/PET Scan

I met with my medical oncologist, Dr. Puhalla, today. The appointment went well; there wasn't anything of concern. Everything looks stable on my CT/PET scans. We are going to yearly tests rather than every 6 months. I am all in favor of this because I get so sick from all the crap they put in my body. We talked about my decision not to take anything when I am finished with the Tamoxifen. Though I know she is very hesitant to go along with it, she is supportive of my decision. I explained that I am aware of the risks, but I want to be "normal" again. Now that it has been five years since my diagnosis, I will only see her once per year, but I can see her more often if I like. I think I will probably go with two times per year.

Wednesday, July 25, 2012
Celebrations!

Bud and I celebrated our first wedding anniversary on July 16th. We went to North Carolina to spend some time with his family since his parents recently moved down there. It was pleasant and relaxing. Since paper is the traditional first anniversary, I asked for dirty green paper...all I got was a dollar! LOL.

Yesterday, I reached another milestone in my cancer journey. I took my last dose of Tamoxifen!! YAY!! One-thousand, eight-hundred and twenty-five doses of this stuff down that hatch! I can hardly believe that I have made it through all five years of taking Tamoxifen. Though I am a bit nervous about not being on it anymore, I am excited for the side effects to go away, and I am hopeful that the pain will also away.

Monday, August 20, 2012
Radiation is the Gift that Keeps on Giving

I went to see my plastic surgeon, Dr. Gimbel, on August 9th, for my yearly follow-up appointment. I was saddened to learn that my favorite nurse, Judy, had retired in January. She happened to be filling in at the office on the day I was there. She was so excited to see me and I, of course, was as happy to see her. The appointment was pretty quick and easy, and despite the outcome, there were no tears shed. Dr. Gimbel checked both implants and noticed what I have been seeing for the past few months...increased dimpling on my right side. He is speculating that this is from the radiation continuing to do its magic. Radiation- it is the gift that keeps on giving. It is not overly noticeable unless you are staring at my chest and depending on what I wear...or, maybe it is, but no one has been brave enough to tell me that it is noticeable.

My shirts and my bras more often than not, end up shifting over to the right side, making me look lopsided. It drives me crazy. With the increased dimpling, I will have to undergo another surgery on the right side to try to fix the dimpling, and I will be getting another implant. When we were talking about my implants and trying to figure out if I had swapped out both the last time, I told Dr. Gimbel that I know for sure both implants had been swapped out. I know this because I have my previous implants in my freezer at home. The hospital was going to get rid of them and called to see if I wanted them; I absolutely did. Dr. Gimbel looked at me a bit sideways, not sure if he had heard me correctly. I laughed and said, "I hope that really doesn't surprise you." I told him that I use them when someone needs a cold com"breast" (rather than a cold compress). He didn't seem to find it as funny as I do. I didn't tell him that I had used them for that purpose when the hub sprained his ankle. True story!!! I will undergo surgery on September 21st, which is a bit sooner than I had hoped, but it is what it is. I go this Friday from my pre-op appointment with my regular physician...Ugh! Surgery is around the corner.

On a much lighter note, I am getting excited about my trip to Disney this coming week with Bud and my youngest niece, Calie. We will be there for seven days, and I have lots of things planned for her. I haven't taken much of a vacation this year, so I am looking forward to this!!

Thursday, September 20, 2012
Stable but Elevated

My gynecological oncologist, Dr. Zorn, called this week to let me know that my CA-125 levels continue to be elevated. They are at 58. She said, "they are consistently elevated but stable, but elevated." The recommendation is to have surgery. Um...no!

September 29, 2012
Breast Reconstruction Surgery

I had my breast reconstruction surgery on Friday, September 21st. My right side had significant dimpling, probably a continued side effect from the radiation. I had to be at Shadyside Hospital by 9:15 am, and surgery was scheduled for 11:15 am. I had my traditional night before surgery Reese's Cup at about 11:30 pm on Thursday. I was up until midnight and got up around 7:00 am.

We got to the hospital and went to the ambulatory surgery center. I was taken back fairly quickly to get ready for surgery. I turned on the tv and watched everything that was happening with the hostage situation in downtown Pittsburgh. The nurse came in to get me ready and to put my IV in place. I told her that I am a hard stick- if she thinks she cannot get me on the first try, I would ask that she get someone else to try. She looked at my veins and was definitely in agreement. I told her that of course, it is my luck that I ended up with a disease that requires being stabbed with needles. She said I should have gotten a port installed, but they only do that when you have chemotherapy. It would be so much easier if they put in a port to access my veins. Anyways, I sat for about five minutes slapping the top of my right hand to wake up my veins to make it easier for the nurse to insert the IV. Silly me...she was putting it on the left side since I was having surgery on the right! UGH!

The anesthetist came in to chat with me before the procedure. I told him I have a hard time coming out from anesthesia. I asked if there is any research to show that repeated exposure to anesthesia causes any changes to brain functions. Sadly, they only suspect that it is safe. Somehow, we ended up talking about concussions. He shared with me that he had sustained a concussion in a quad accident with his son and had to be off work for several months. After I signed consent for the anesthesia, I had my IV put in. The nurse started to use a butterfly but then decided to go smaller because my veins are so tiny. I was so thankful. She said they could change it while I was under if needed. Why am I only learning this now?

After I was all prepped for surgery, they brought Bud in to be with me. I waited about a half-hour before Dr. Gimbel came in and marked the right side. A short time later, they gave me a happy drug through my IV and was wheeled off to surgery. I don't know precisely how long the procedure took. I don't remember much of being in the recovery room, the step-down recovery, the ride home, or the rest of the night. I was more out of it after this surgery than any other I have had.

I do recall being in the recovery room, and the nurse asked me about my pain. I remember not being able to open my eyes or talk. I gave her a thumbs up to indicate that I was in lots of pain. Luckily, she was able to figure that out. I recall a short time after that I felt like I was going to vomit. I started yelling, "I am going to be sick; I am going to be sick." I never opened my eyes. Someone came over to my bedside, and I started to vomit. I threw up twice and then was done. I think I passed out for a time, but when I woke up, I felt sick again. I still couldn't open my eyes, but I could hear the nurse talking to the lady they had just brought in about how she was very coherent and came out of the anesthesia so fast. Gosh, I wish that were me! I started yelling again that I was going to be sick. No one was around, but thankfully, the lady next to me told her nurse that I was going to get sick. I wish I could have thanked her for that. Again, someone came over and sure enough, I started to vomit. I was freaked out because I have never gotten sick while in recovery. I was out quickly after another dose of anti-nausea medication.

I vaguely remember them wheeling me out of recovery to step-down recovery. I was transferred from the bed to a chair. I don't know how long I was in step-down recovery and I don't remember much about being in step-down recovery. Apparently, I asked Bud for my umbrella and was concerned that he would forget it at the hospital. The nurse said I asked for it in the recovery room as well. Um...okay. I did not bring an umbrella with me. When I left the hospital, I was completely incoherent. I am shocked that they let me go home. Given the state I was in, I know they shouldn't have let me leave the hospital. Bud told me that they put me in a wheelchair, someone took me down to the garage area, they got me into the car, and Bud and I headed home. We stopped to get my antibiotic, but I don't remember that either. We got home, and I was out the rest of the night.

When I woke up the next day and was slightly more coherent, but I was in a good bit of pain. I took the Vicodin until Tuesday or Wednesday and was taking two at a time. This is totally not like me at all! I have been sore all week, have lots of bruising, and am sensitive to the touch. All things considered, the right side looks pretty good. However, it appears as though I am lopsided. I don't know if this is because I am swollen or if I really am lopsided. I have 500cc on the right side and 425cc on the left side, so I'm guessing there is some lopsidedness. UGH! I did tell Dr. Gimbel that he should swap out the left side too, but he didn't think that was necessary...we shall discuss when I see him on Thursday. My range of motion is not very good, which means I will probably have to do physical therapy AGAIN. I hate PT. I did try stretching my arm, but the pain was excruciating, and I had to take more pain medication.

I discovered that sneezing and laughing HURT! I haven't experienced that since my mastectomy and the expanders. I'm guessing it is because my chest is somewhat tight. I was watching The Ellen DeGeneres Show on

Friday and thought my incision had split open because I was laughing so hard.

I go back to work on Monday. I am okay with that because I am bored out of my mind. I am not allowed to lift anything over ten pounds for eight weeks and am not allowed to exercise other than light walking for that time. Bummer!

The downside of surgery is that Bud is not a great cook, so I am left to my own devices for feeding myself. He actually brought me Chipotle on Monday...yeah, that almost came back up. I don't say anything because I know he is trying the best he can, but he is awful at it. Luckily, one of my friends brought us stuff for dinner one day.

After having my eighth surgery and constantly feeling so out of shape, I have decided that I am going to run my first marathon in February 2014. It is the Disney Princess Half Marathon. I think I am going to get a group of people together to do the marathon, including my medical oncologist! How fun!!

Friday, January 4, 2013
Lopsided Foobies

I have been doing an online class on brain injury this past semester that just about sucked the life right out of me...and it was only an intro class. I was able to get through the course and ended up with an A Woo Hoo. However, I have been slacking on my journaling as a result.

I saw my plastic surgeon, Dr. Gimbel, in October for my six-week follow-up. The appointment was fairly uneventful. He checked my incisions, and everything looked good though I was still obviously very bruised. I talked with him about my obvious lopsidedness. I have to wait until my next appointment before we had any further discussion about that because he seemed to think that I was still swollen and that with time, I should even out nicely. The next several months were relatively uneventful except for what I called cancer-induced meltdowns. With it being winter time, being able to wear sweaters is pretty much my saving grace for others to not notice how lopsided I am, but we had several days when it was warmer outside and that caused my meltdowns. I put on shirt after shirt after shirt and everything shifted over to the right side. Not a little...a lot and everything was shifted including the neckline of my shirts. I cried because I couldn't hide it. Thankfully that only happened twice but when it did happen it was pretty bad.

In December, I saw my radiation oncologist, Dr. Beriwal, for what I expected to be the last time. Typically, when people hit the five-year mark, they are released. I was yet again happy but nervous that I would no longer be under the watchful eye of my radiation oncologist. My appointment was as it typically is...short and uneventful, but Dr. Beriwal said, "okay, we will see you in one year." Um...oh...ok. Not that I was all that disappointed but was totally not expecting that.

I returned to see my plastic surgeon, Dr. Gimbel, yesterday. Since I continue to be lopsided, I anticipated that the appointment would include a discussion about another surgery, but that was never even brought up. He came in and examined me and seemed to think that everything was fine. I shared with him that I am concerned about being lopsided with one side being more prominent than the other and told him that my shirts keep shifting. Much to my dismay, there probably isn't much more that can be done. He says that I am not bigger on one side than the other even though my right implant is 500cc and the left side is 425cc. It seems logical to me that in fact, one side is larger than the other.

I tried explaining it to him but was in tears because he was telling me that I need to consider changing the clothing I wear. I think I looked at him with rage in my eyes because I'm talking about sweaters and t-shirts. I'm not talking about shirts that show off my chest. Then he said, "well, can't

312

you find a bra to fix that." I chuckled at him and said, I cannot even find a bra that works. I have been searching for over five years now and haven't found anything. My bra shifts over to the right side too. I was also getting pissed off because he repeatedly said, "I understand." I wanted to scream at him and say, "No, you don't. You cannot even possibly begin to understand." At one point, he closed the robe I was wearing and said, "well, this isn't shifting." I said, "Of course, it isn't shifting, it is a robe." According to him, I have to learn to live with it. I told him that he will have to show me how to do that because I will not simply live with it. I left there so angry and upset. I hadn't gotten any further in my discussion with him about being lopsided. I couldn't even talk with him through all of the tears. I made an appointment to go back in March with several shirts in hand to show him what I am talking about since he clearly does not see the problem. I'm not looking to be perfect because I know that will never happen, but I am NOT okay with being lopsided!!!

Friday, January 11, 2013
Clean Ovarian Screening, Finally!

I went to see my gynecological oncologist, Dr. Zorn on Friday, January 5th. I had both the ultrasound and my CA-125 levels checked. They found an endometrial polyp, which should go away with my next monthly visit from Charlie. There were no cysts, nothing at all on my ovaries. NOTHING AT ALL! That never happens. I called this week to find out what my CA-125 levels were and much to my surprise and excitement, they dropped to 46 from 58. It is still elevated but down by twelve points. That is huge. The only things I have changed since my last appointment are that I am now under the care of a chiropractor for better overall health, and I have started eating healthy and cleaner (pretty much vegan). I am in complete and total shock that it has gone down and by that much. My levels have been in the upper 50's/lower 60's range for two years. I am so happy.

I have an appointment scheduled with my medical oncologist, Dr. Puhalla, for February 22nd. I expect that we will talk about me going back on Tamoxifen. A study was recently released that showed taking ten years of Tamoxifen proves to be more effective than five years of the medication and that five years may actually be dangerous. We shall see what she says.

Monday, February 25, 2013
Tamoxifen Revisited

On February 22nd, I had my yearly visit with Dr. Puhalla, my medical oncologist. It was a rather lengthy visit this time. I was checked by the fellow and then seen by Dr. Puhalla. There was nothing of concern on the exam, as usual. I did talk to her at length about my apparent lopsidedness, and she indicated that she can clearly see that the right side is protruding out further than the left side. I showed her several photos that I had taken of me in different shirts, and she was taken back by the fact that it is so apparent in my clothing. She did explain to me that this may be the best that Dr. Gimbel can do with getting the foobies to be symmetrical and said that even though to the rest of the world, 425cc is less than 500cc, it may not truly be. Apparently, in the field of plastic surgery, they have their own math that only they can understand. All I know is that regardless of whether it is plastic surgeon math or regular math, at the end of the day, I am lopsided and not okay with it.

We also talked about the one thing I was dreading the most...Tamoxifen. I was hoping that we wouldn't be having that conversation but no such luck. She would like for me to go back on Tamoxifen for another 5 years based on the results of the study that were released in San Antonio Breast Cancer Symposium this past year. In short, this study suggests that ten years of Tamoxifen is more effective in reducing recurrence and death. Previous studies suggested that five years was sufficient.

Considering that I am BRCA2 positive and given that Dr. Puhalla wanted me to switch to a different medication following the Tamoxifen, she feels very strongly that I should go back on the Tamoxifen. She said that they hope to keep me alive until I am at least 80 years old and I told her there is no reason to get all crazy! I asked for the prescription for Tamoxifen to have on hand, but I have not yet filled it. Now that I think of it, I don't even know where it is. I did tell her that I wanted to talk with my nutritionist about it to get her opinion, and Dr. Puhalla agreed.

It has taken me way too long to figure out that there is truth in the saying- "Let thy food by thy medicine, and thy medicine be thy food." Eating better has significantly changed my life even though I didn't eat all that horribly before. I did talk with my nutritionist at my last visit. She suggested I increase my intake of broccoli, kale, cauliflower, and cabbage...every single day. She also put me on a new supplement called cruciferous complete, which includes something called DIM. From what I have read, DIM is like Tamoxifen but is healthier as it comes from a chemical compound found in cruciferous vegetables. Though there is little research on the actual benefits of DIM related to cancer, it is suspected that it may be effective against breast cancer. My nutritionist is going to order a urine test for me that will determine how my body breaks down hormones. This will help with the decision of going back on the Tamoxifen. It is not covered by insurance, but it seems well worth it to know how my body reacts to hormones and let my decision be guided by that. I did ask my nutritionist why this test would not be used in conventional medical facilities to help guide individual treatment, and she said that her guess was as good as mine.

I will have my yearly PET/CT scan scheduled within the next few months, and I am back to visits with Dr. Puhalla every six months rather than every year.

I also learned at my appointment with Dr. Puhalla that my gynecological oncologist at Hillman, Dr. Zorn, is relocating to Texas. I was in complete shock and felt lost. I have worked closely with Dr. Zorn for the past six years now, and we developed a close and trusting relationship. That is hard to let go of. I hate the thought of having to find another gynecological oncologist. All of the other doctors in that office are males. Nothing against male doctors but they don't have the understanding of girlie parts that a female doctor has.

Monday, March 11, 2013
Lopsided Foobies

I went back to see my plastic surgeon, Dr. Gimbel, on March 7th, to talk about my lopsidedness. He asked that I bring in several different shirts to put on but, who has time for that. I took several photos with my phone to show him what is happening. I prepared myself for the appointment and what I wanted to say in hopes of not becoming emotional. I held up pretty well this time. Initially, he didn't seem to be getting what I was saying. I showed him a picture of me in my bra that ends up more to the right side, but he didn't see that as a significant issue. I do have a problem with the fact that I cannot wear a bra without it shifting. I showed him several other pictures that clearly show my clothing shifting to the right side. I think it finally started to click with him. He had me sit straight up and then looked at the implants from above, which at least from my perspective, shows that I am lopsided. He tried to measure how far out the implant on the right side protrudes in comparison to the left but was unable to do so. According to his handy-dandy chart, they are the same, but after further review, he realized that there is a misprint- the 500cc implant does have more protrusion than the 425cc implant. He used a ruler to attempt to see how much the left side is off from the right side and of course, without the ability to measure perfectly, it is about an inch.

I realize some may not think this is a big deal...one side is usually bigger than the other, but there is clearly a difference between how that difference is observed on natural breasts and the silicone-filled plastic pouches inside my chest. Dr. Gimbel indicated that he can go back in to swap out the implant for a smaller implant with less protrusion but the same volume. He also plans to do more liposuction from the latissimus flap, which is also likely adding some additional protrusion. He did say that if I had enough latissimus muscle, he would have used the while muscle to rebuild the entire breast but because I am so small, it was not an option. I am scheduled to have another surgery on May 10th...the exact same surgery I had in September 2012. I do have very mixed emotions about it. There are days I don't think I want to go through with it, but then there are days when I get so upset when I cannot find a shirt to wear because it shifts t to the right side. Maybe I am being vain, I don't know, but I know I want to feel comfortable with how I look and right now I don't. I certainly hope that this will be the last surgery I have for some time though he was unequivocal in telling me that he cannot guarantee that it will be. Unfortunately, in addition to my lopsidedness, I have noticed that the right implant is "bubbling" under my skin, which I have attributed to the lasting impact of radiation. I had Dr. Gimbel check it out, and he also thinks that it is related to the radiation. Yes, I am now five and a half years out of radiation. I asked him if he thought that I would always be impacted by the radiation, and he said, "yes because it is the gift that keeps on giving." I laughed and told him that I say the same thing all of the time!

Friday, March 15, 2013
Not So Happy Cancerversary

I hadn't intended to write this journal update on my cancerversary and certainly not at 4:30 am, but I woke up at 3:00 am in so much pain from my monthly visitor, Charlie. I am sitting on the couch with my heating pad on my belly and cannot go back to sleep. What else do I have to do but update my journal, right? So here it is...about four hours from now, it will officially be my six-year cancerversary. Six years...I can hardly believe it. Some days I feel like it was yesterday because it is so fresh in my mind, but then other days, it is so distant that it feels like forever ago. I didn't ever imagine I would be where I am today, and on the flip side of that, I didn't ever imagine that I would still be dealing with this. I often wonder if there will be a time in my life that I'm not dealing with something related to cancer. I don't know...I guess at this point in my journey, I don't expect it. I suppose I finally realize that it may never go away, and I need to learn to live with that. It's funny that I remember seeing a pamphlet pretty early on in my journey about learning to live with cancer. I thought that was so silly and didn't have a full understanding of what it meant. After six years of hoping that I wouldn't have to learn to live with cancer...I am... I am trying.

Wednesday, July 10, 2013
New Gynecological Oncologist

I had my bi-annual ovarian cancer screening this week. I met my new gynecological oncologist since Dr. Zorn left Hillman. I wasn't overly impressed with the new doctor...I can't even remember her name. She clearly had not spent any time reading my chart, and all I kept thinking was, "I would never let this woman operate on me."

I did the sonogram and then was taken down to have my blood drawn for the CA-125. I forgot to drink water in the morning, so I asked for some water. Even with that, my veins were nowhere to be found. They had me wrapped in about five blankets and I had a heating pad on each arm. I sat for about then minutes and then finally, I was ready. The nurse was able to draw blood the first time! Woo Hoo!

Friday, July 31, 2013
CA-125 Levels Sky Rocketed

I got a message on my cell phone on Tuesday, July 16th, my second wedding anniversary, from the nurse saying that my CA-125 levels had jumped from 40 something last time to 118.5. She said the doctor wanted to retest in a few weeks. If my levels were still elevated, we would discuss surgery. My heart sank. I so badly wanted my husband at that moment, but I was in the middle of my last class in Washington, D.C., at George Washington University. I went back to class and was clearly teary-eyed. My friend Gina took me out into the hallway. When I told her about the phone message, she put her arms around me and hugged me.

I sent a few text messages to Bud, and he said, be happy...today is our anniversary. I was happy about that, but I was also sad because I was not home with him. I got through the rest of my class that day. As I was standing on Gina's front porch, where I was staying for the week, I heard someone behind us asking for directions. It took a second for it to register, but I knew it was Bud. He had driven down to D.C. so that we could celebrate our anniversary. We ate dinner at the Lafayette and stayed the night at the Adams Hotel. They gave us a complimentary upgrade for our room, which faced the White House, and also gave us a cake and a bottle of champagne. It was amazing! He is amazing!

I had my retest done a week or so after getting back from D.C., and my levels had dropped down to 46. I was elated!

Sunday, September 22, 2013
May 2013 Surgery

This journal entry is well overdue. I had intended to write this following my surgery in May, but there are so many emotions surrounding that time that I couldn't bring myself to write this. Four months later, there is still a lot of emotion, but I feel like I am somewhat ready to write this.

On May 10th, I underwent another reconstructive surgery to fix the right implant. I wasn't sure that I was going to go through with this surgery until the last minute. Two days before my surgery, my younger brother had a traumatic accident.

When I received the call from my mother, I only remember throwing my shoes on, asking my husband if he was going, telling him he could drive, but then deciding to drive myself because we would get there faster. I don't know how fast I was going, but I beat the ambulance to the hospital. I was standing there as they pulled my brother out of the back of the ambulance and lost it. I ran into the emergency entrance behind the EMT but was stopped by a nurse.

It seemed to take forever for my parents and older brother to arrive. While we were waiting for them, the nurse informed me that my brother would be transferred to another hospital. We were ready to leave right as my parents and older brother pulled into the parking lot. I led the caravan to Allegheny General Hospital, and once again, we beat the ambulance. We were in the public waiting room briefly before the staff put us in a private waiting area. Emotions were high, and we sat in complete silence. We were expecting the worst. It felt like hours had passed before someone finally came back to talk with us. After waiting another hour, we were taken up to the intensive care unit waiting room. We were permitted to see him, but I just stood outside the door. I was very stoic on the outside, but inside I was falling apart. I couldn't imagine losing my younger brother.

After talking with the doctors again, we went back outside into the waiting area. I started calling and texting family members and friends to give them an update. At about 4:00 am, I left to take Bud home and to get ready to go to work. I never slept that night; I went home and cleaned my house until it was time to go to work. It was apparent that I had not slept, and my boss kept telling me to go home. I had several things that I needed to get done before I could leave. My surgery was the following day, and I would be out for two weeks. I was able to finish everything and left mid-morning. I went home to change and then headed back to the hospital. Bud joined us at the hospital around noon. We ate lunch and dinner at the hospital. At around 5:00 pm, Bud suggested that we get home so that I could get some rest before my surgery in the morning. I didn't want to leave my family in the middle of all of what was going on, but the doctor assured me that my brother would make a full recovery and it would be okay for me to go forward with my surgery.

That evening Dr. Gimbel, my plastic surgeon, called me and asked me to come a little later in the day for my surgery. I do prefer to be scheduled super early rather than mid-morning because I'm usually starving at that point and would seriously eat anything. I willingly complied.

We arrived at the hospital close to 10:00 am. The typical sequence of events occurred. They took me up alone, prepped me for surgery, and then let Bud join me. I took a picture of myself in my hospital gown and sent it to my older brother to show my younger brother. I said, "tell him we are twins." When the anesthesiologist arrived, I talked with him about my issues with vomiting after surgery. He said that they would change things so that I wouldn't be so sick. I forgot to tell my plastic surgeon, Dr. Gimbel, of my recent allergic reaction to surgical tape though. The surgery went well and was pretty fast. I was put into my own personal recovery room rather than with the general population.

Though the anesthesiologist assured me that I wouldn't be as sick, I was much worse than during my last surgery. I threw up multiple times. I tried ice chips, but that came back up. Crackers...came back up. Sprite...came back up. Nothing was staying down. Since I was vomiting, my pain medications were coming back up too. I was miserable. After several hours, I got the impression that it was the end of the nurse's shift, so I was being pressured to leave. I needed another dosage of pain medication, but that meant, I would have to stay longer. They hooked me up with a blanket, pillow, and several vomit buckets before sending us out the door. We arrived home, and I was still miserable. I didn't try to eat anything for the rest of the evening.

Saturday brought with it the most horrific experience I have ever had following surgery. I vomited up everything I tried to consume. I was in so much pain because I was vomiting. I was also having a severe allergic reaction to the surgical tape. I was absolutely miserable. I went through all of Saturday feeling like this. I had posted something on Facebook and many friends suggested that I go back to the hospital. I wasn't doing that. I waited it out and called Dr. Gimbel at 5:00 am on Sunday. I was told that he wouldn't get the message until 7:00 am. I waited and waited but never heard from him. I remembered that he had called my cell phone the night before my surgery, so I had his personal cell number and called him. He was not informed that I called the messaging system. He was upset that he didn't get the message and was not called immediately. Dr. Gimbel sent over a prescription for anti-nausea medication, and Bud was able to get it by mid-morning on Sunday. I continued to take it for several days to control nausea.

322

Bud also picked up some Benadryl to help with the allergic reaction. The combination of the anti-nausea medication and the Benadryl knocked me out. I slept more during this recovery than any other. I went for my follow-up appointment, and Dr. Gimbel was pleased. More importantly, so was I. He was concerned with the allergic reaction to the tape as I saw him two and a half weeks post-surgery and was still having issues. He removed the tape that was left behind and asked that I come back if the reaction didn't resolve. I was very itchy for a few weeks after but couldn't take any Benadryl because I was back to work and Benadryl me out. The allergic reaction did eventually resolve. I need to remember to share that I am allergic to surgical tape next time...if there is a next time.

Currently, I am feeling great. I am training for the Disney Princess Half Marathon on February 23rd in Disney World. I am not a runner and haven't been able to get back on track with working out for the past six years with all of the surgeries, but I am determined to do this. We will leave for Disney on February 20th, which is the anniversary of finding my lump and then I will run on the 23rd. I cannot think of any better way to say "Fuck you" to cancer. I have two friends that will be joining me as well as my medical oncologist, Dr. Puhalla. I am totally geeked over it!

Tuesday, February 19, 2014
The Unavoidable Pelvic Sweep

I saw my new gynecological oncologist at the beginning of February, and we talked at great length about the unavoidable full pelvic sweep. I was a bit uncomfortable initially and still continue to be unimpressed by her...she doesn't even know enough about me to know that I have a history of breast cancer. Through our discussion, I learned that she would not be the one to perform the surgery, much to my relief. Dr. Mansuria, my gynecological specialist, will be conducting the operation.

My plan at the time of that conversation was to schedule the surgery for May 2015; however, there is a dispute between Highmark Blue Cross, Blue Shield and the University of Pittsburgh Medical Center (UPMC). I may be forced to seek out new providers beginning January 1, 2015 or have the surgery before that. All of my doctors are at UPMC, so this is a bit unsettling to me. I talked with the finance guy at work on Friday about what will happen if Highmark and UPMC cannot come to an agreement. He indicated that he is hopeful that a resolution will be made, but it will probably take place at the eleventh hour. If there is no resolution, we will not immediately change insurance companies. This means I will either have to change all of my doctors or I can continue to be seen by UPMC, but it will be out of network and that can become very costly. So as of right now, I have decided that I will move that surgery up to December 2014. GASP!!! I cannot take the risk of not having this surgery covered by my insurance or having to put my trust in a doctor that I don't have any kind of relationship with. This has thrown me off a bit...I was mentally preparing myself for it to be next spring. It won't be easy for me no matter when I do it, but I felt like spring would have been great because I will be two months from turning 40, and well, that is beyond the age I should be considering having a child, right? Maybe...maybe not but it was what I was going with in hopes of making it easier. I cry any time I think about the fact that I will never have a child...hell, I am crying now. I am terrified of the emotional mess that I will be when that becomes final.

Tuesday, February 26, 2014
Disney Princess Half Marathon

I completed the Disney Princess Half Marathon on February 23rd. It was pretty awesome to have a great team of supporters there with me, including my medical oncologist, Dr. Puhalla. The whole experience was over the top, and I am glad that my first half marathon was in Disney. It was harder than I expected. I trained well for it, but I made it to the end. Honestly, I didn't care if I ran, walked, or crawled...as long as I finished. I pushed myself harder than I have ever pushed myself to complete it. Not finishing wasn't even an option.

Sadly, I found out that morning, my fellow breast cancer survivor, Vanessa, had passed away. I was crushed. Vanessa and I were both diagnosed on March 15, 2007. She was only in her 20's when diagnosed. Her journey was long and hard, but Vanessa never lost her will to keep fighting. She started the Live Sincerely Project (www.thelivesincerelyproject.com), asking that everyone take the pledge to live sincerely each and every day. Even though Vanessa is no longer here with us and will be sadly missed, her spirit lives on through her project. Please take the pledge today and live your life sincerely every single day...you never know when it might be your last.

Tuesday, May 14, 2014
Health and Happiness

Wow! Time does fly by when you are having fun. I cannot believe that I reached my seven-year cancerversary mark on March 15th and didn't even write about it!

Bud and I started off 2014 with a goal to get healthy. As of today, he is down about sixty pounds, and I lost the weight I have gained since we got married. We are the healthiest and happiest we have ever been in our lives. We continue to work on renovating our house and are close to being finished. We have been tossing around the idea of moving to Arizona in the near future. I have gotten back into dragon boating and will be traveling to Sarasota, FL to participate in international competition.

Wednesday, September 25, 2014
Surgery is Scheduled

I am scheduled to have my next, and hopefully last, major surgery on November 11, 2014, at Passavant Hospital. Dr. Mansuria will do a full pelvic sweep- removing my ovaries, uterus, and fallopian tubes. *VOMIT* My recovery time is expected to be four weeks. I am not looking forward to it, but the good thing is that I have been busy with work and dragon boating that I don't have any time to even think about it! This will be a tough recovery time for me simply because I won't be able to sit out in my sunroom as I have the past several surgeries because it will be cold and snowy, and Bud will not be home every day to take care of me...he is now working outside of the house.

Monday, November 11, 2014
Surgery Day is Here

I planned to get up this morning and write in my journal about this one topic I have avoided for so long, but they have bumped up my surgery by an hour. I will be leaving here to go to the hospital in a few moments. I guess this is a good thing because I have pushed all of this out of my mind and haven't allowed myself to deal with it. I hope that I don't lose it when I am there. I am not ready for this...I have never been ready for this. I don't know that I will ever be ready for it, but it is here, and there is no turning back at this point. My surgery is at 11:00 am.

Monday, December 16, 2014
Goodbye Ovaries, Goodbye Fallopian Tubes, Goodbye Uterus

It is currently five weeks post-surgery as of today. I can hardly believe that much time has passed and I still have not found it in myself to write this entry. Of all the things I have dealt with over the past seven years, I have struggled the most with having the total hysterectomy and oophorectomy. To be honest, I can't say that I was still even ready for it when I had the surgery done. The issue was forced upon me, given the current dispute between Highmark and UPMC. Having the operation covered by insurance and done by Dr. Mansuria meant that it had to be done before January 1, 2015. Good thing patients come first.

I had scheduled the surgery back in July knowing that with dragon boating season in full swing, I wouldn't have much time to think about the operation. I kept myself occupied every single day from the day I had scheduled it until the day leading up to the surgery. It was the only way I knew I would be able to get through it. I had dragon boating practice three to four times per week, but as the international competition got closer, we were practicing five to six days per week. It was probably the best distraction I had. On a side note, we went to Sarasota, Florida at the end of October. There were over a hundred teams from all around the world, and we came in 2nd place in the world and 1st place in the United States. How freaking awesome is that?!?!?

November 11th came pretty quickly after getting home from Sarasota. My surgery was scheduled for 10:00 am, but then they called me later in the day on the 10th to tell me it has been pushed back to noon. I was frustrated because I prefer to have my surgery first thing in the morning, and I was on a liquid diet that had started after my huge breakfast. That meant twenty-four hours of water, chicken broth, and Jell-O. I didn't even get to have my traditional Reese's Cup at midnight. The day before was pretty uneventful but being home alone and not being able to eat was dreadful. I got up on the morning of the 11th a few minutes before my phone rang. It was a nurse telling me that my surgery had been bumped up to 11:00 am instead of noon. We rushed to get ready and over to the hospital. We sat in the waiting room for almost a half-hour before I was taken into pre-op. Bud and I sat there anxiously waiting. I laid my head upon his chest, and he wrapped his arm around me as tears streamed down my face. I covered myself with the Pink Steel blanket my teammates had gotten for me. A lady sat down across from us and started to eat her sandwich. I swear I was so hungry that I wanted to steal it from her and devour it even though it looked to be a ham sandwich. Who eats a ham sandwich at 9:00 am in the morning, anyways??

I was happy when they finally called me back to go into pre-op. After ten previous surgeries, it is like a walk in the park for me at this point. They were able to get my IV in on the first try, which made my day. I laid there with my Pink Steel blanket and my jersey from Sarasota that all of my teammates had signed for me. The nurse was great, and she seemed to enjoy hearing all about my trip to Sarasota.

When the anesthesiologist came into the room, I talked with him at length about my most recent surgery- how horrible it was coming out of anesthesia and getting horribly sick after. He decided that he would give me an anti-nausea medication beforehand and put a patch behind my ear to also help with nausea. I was hopeful that maybe I wouldn't be so bad off this time around. Two other doctors had come into the room to answer any questions I had. I didn't have any questions. I quietly cried as they explained the surgery to me. I could see that the nurse was watching and had a hard time holding back her own tears. Dr. Mansuria came into the room and asked if I had any questions. He told me that he had to initial my ovaries, which made me laugh hysterically. He told me not to laugh because it is so silly that he has to do it, but I did laugh...and loudly. Bud entered the room soon after, and I told him that Dr. Mansuria had initialed my ovaries. He giggled about that as well. It was only about fifteen minutes before Dr. Mansuria came back in to let me know that they were ready. Bud kissed me. As they wheeled me out, I cried. Through the blur of my tears, I saw Bud standing against the wall mouthing the words "I love you" to me. I said, "I love you too." I was wheeled into the operating room and was out shortly after.

The surgery took about two hours, maybe two and a half. When I came to in the recovery room, I had a lot of pain. I wasn't expecting to be in as much pain as I was. The nurse was doing everything she could to keep me comfortable. She was alternating between pain medication and anti-nausea medication, both of which knocked me completely out. I woke up at one point and asked for something to throw up in. She handed me a green bag with a plastic rim. She gave me some more anti-nausea medication, and thankfully, I never threw up. I recall a doctor coming over, looking at me, and saying, "Oh yea, she is green." I said, "I am green? Like Elphaba green?" He giggled and told me that I was green, as in I looked nauseous. I fell back to sleep. I was coming in and out of consciousness, which made the nurse very uncomfortable and worried. I have no idea how many times she called Bud to give him an update, but it was a lot. Dr. Mansuria came in at one point and sat down on my bed. He said the surgery had gone well. He then said, "So you have been working on your abs, huh?" I laughed and said, "yes." He told me to keep up the great job because they look great. I told him my goal was for them to notice my abs. I was out again quickly after that brief conversation.

The nurse had decided that it was best to keep me overnight because she could not get a handle on the pain and nausea. She told me that she was giving me baby doses of each, but it was still knocking me out. She told me to be sure to start drinking alcohol to help my tolerance for the anesthesia and pain medications in the future. Typically, caregivers are not permitted to go back into the recovery room, but she said she had called for Bud to come back and be with me until they could get me into a room. I had been in recovery for about five hours before she called for him. We were there another two before they finally got me in a room. Right before they moved me, I had to use the bathroom. In my mind, I thought I would be able to walk the short distance from my bed to the bathroom, but that was not the case. Two of the nurses wheeled me into the bathroom on the bed. I tried to swing my legs over the bed to stand up, but as soon as I tried that, I shrieked in pain. I had to roll onto my side and then sit up, stand, and walk over to the toilet. Holy shit did that hurt!! I finished in the bathroom, got back in the bed, and they wheeled me back out.

I was transported to my room and transferred from the gurney onto the bed. For me, that is one of the worst parts. It was painful, as it always is, but not the worst I have experienced. I got settled in and told Bud to go home because I know that sleeping in a hospital chair is very uncomfortable and we only live about fifteen minutes away. I slept through most of the night, except they woke me up almost every hour to check my vitals. I woke in the morning and ordered breakfast. The nurse came in to give me my medication. She forced me to take the Tamoxifen even though I told her I wouldn't be taking it anymore. It wasn't worth arguing about. I was excited that they finally gave me a pair of undies and a pad. I was bleeding internally, as would be expected, and they simply put a large absorbent pad under me and let me bleed. UGH! I was able to get up from the bed with some help, go to the bathroom, and get cleaned up. I was dressed and ready to go by the time Bud got there. I finished my breakfast, had my IVs taken out, and was out the door.

I didn't do much for the first four weeks of my recovery. I stopped taking the meds pretty quickly because I hate taking medication. I slept on the chaise for almost two-and-a-half weeks because getting out of bed was too painful. I immediately had a reaction to the band-aids and the surgical glue. I had four incisions- one in my bellybutton, near each of my hip bones, and then one incision near my pelvic bone. When I removed the band-aid from my lower incision, I had popped one blister, but there was another blister. For three weeks, I was so itchy, and I was seeping from the blisters that had developed under the glue. I finally called Dr. Mansuria's office and asked if I can pull the glue off. The nurse was baffled that I am allergic to the glue and band-aids. She asked me what I typically do. I told her that I take Benadryl, but that knocks me out. She talked with Dr. Mansuria, and he thought it would be okay to take the glue off. Of course, the itchiness was even worse after I had removed the glue. Go figure!

Bud took me out to dinner a few times to keep me from going crazy but not for too long, as I was exhausted after only a short time. I had many visitors. I got to see my Uncle Warren, who lives in Arizona and finally got to see my two youngest nieces after almost a year. I kept myself occupied by reading a book that a dear friend bought for me, writing letters, and writing sponsorship letters for Pink Steel. The week of Thanksgiving, I spoke at the Pitt Medical Conference, as I do every year. On Thanksgiving, we delivered dinner to cancer survivors through Cancer Fighting Princess. We had four families this year and thankfully had volunteers to help. There was an article in the Pittsburgh Post-Gazette the day before, and we were on the news on Thanksgiving Day. It was wonderful!

I went for my follow-up appointment with Dr. Mansuria on Monday, December 8th. It was probably the fastest appointment I have ever had. He was in there for less than five minutes, seriously! He told me that all went well. They found two spots of endometriosis, which have been removed. He took out the remaining stitches from my bellybutton and my lower incision, and then he was gone. I went back to work on Wednesday, December 11th. I was swollen like a balloon and in pain by the end of the day. I went in on Thursday and Friday but was still swollen and in pain. Several of my friends commented on how swollen my tummy was. I called Dr. Mansuria, who suggested I take Monday and Tuesday off this week and then return for half days until school is on winter break.

Interestingly, everyone I have talked to said that they were off for six to eight weeks, but yet I was released at four weeks. Initially, Dr. Mansuria wasn't going to give me the time off, but I pushed for it. When I talked to the nurse, I told her that I am incredibly disappointed that my perspective as a patient was not being considered. I hadn't been swollen and wasn't in pain for several days, but with returning to work and walking so much, I was. I told her that to me, my body is telling me to slow down and that it is not ready. I explained that I would not be calling her if I weren't having a lot of pain because I am not one to complain about pain. Honestly, I don't understand what difference it makes how much time I take off. It isn't like Dr. Mansuria is cutting my paycheck, and my boss is super supportive of me.

I am now menopausal. Yea that is completed fucked up. I didn't have many symptoms during the first week. Then it hit me! I have had hot flashes when taking the Tamoxifen, but this was different. It felt like a match had been lit and was burning from the inside out. I was getting them ALOT!! Then the night sweats started, which were even worse. I was tossing and turning as I slept because I was so hot. I would push everything off of me, and sometimes take off all of my night clothes to cool down. Sweat was dripping off of me like I had completed the most intense workout ever. And then, I was freezing again. I had to put everything back on, cover myself up, and then it happened all over again.

At the recommendation of Dr. Puhalla, my medical oncologist, I started taking Vitamin E twice a day, which seems to help some. I still have hot flashes and night sweats here and there though but not as intense as before. I hear that other symptoms come along with menopause, but I am still waiting for those. We shall see how this goes. I am now taking Arimidex to continue to lower the level of estrogen in my body. I haven't had many side effects from that yet. It made me dizzy the first week or so that I had taken it, but that seems to have stopped.

I still haven't dealt with the hardest part of all of this, and I am not sure when or if I will. I have pushed it into the back of my head and kept it out of my heart. I know it is there; every so often it starts to creep up, but I push it back again. I make jokes about it with Bud at times because laughter and humor are my best coping mechanisms.

Maybe the day will come that I will deal with it, perhaps it won't.

Interested in More?

Check out the official **Behind** the **Pink Ribbon** podcast.

Download & Subscribe Today

Available on Apple Podcasts or Google Podcasts, as well as many other podcasting apps like Stitcher, Spreaker, Pandora, and iHeartRadio!

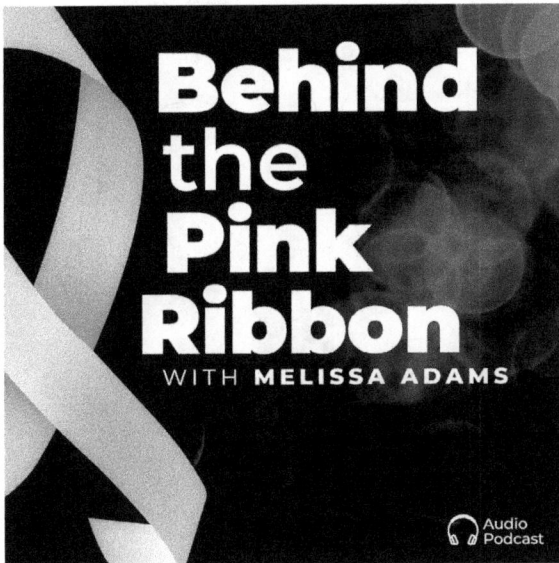

Visit the show online at:
www.BehindthePinkRibbon.com

ISBN: 978-1-7340803-0-8 (Paperback)

Library of Congress Control Number: 2019914724

Front cover image by Bud Adams.
Book design by American Creative Consulting.

Printed by Amazon KDP, in the United States of America.

First printing edition 2019.

American Creative Consulting
1023 W Ingram St.
Mesa, AZ 85201

www.behindthepinkribbon.com
www.americancreativeconsulting.com